Living Well in Body, Mind, and Spirit

By Dr. Brian Kovara

∞

Life Design Publishing

ISBN-13: 978-1987658668

ISBN-10: 1987658663

TABLE OF CONTENTS

Greetings and Welcome!

Chiropractic care is the practice of using spinal alignment to alleviate a wide variety of physical ailments, including muscle strain, neck pain, chronic back pain, and more. This is accomplished by adjusting the position of the spinal column to its proper shape, providing a non-invasive solution for pain relief.

My name is Dr. Brian Kovara and I've been a Doctor of Chiropractic (DC) since 2000. My wife April and our family moved to this area in 2014. If you're looking for a chiropractor, I hope we can meet. Choosing a health care provider is a big decision.

At Living Well Chiropractic & Massage we believe that education is a big part of our patients' success so have dedicated this entire website to helping you understand the full scope of what our team can do for you as you work to meet your wellness goals.

The vast majority of people equate chiropractic with back pain, but the circumstances under which the science of Chiropractic Care was discovered, at that time, had little to do with back pain.

The founder of chiropractic care, Daniel David ("D.D.") Palmer, believed that many conditions could be addressed by removing pressure from the nerve that was involved with the affected area. He proceeded to make his life's work about turning this belief into the science of chiropractic. Palmer called it "a science of healing without drugs."

Chiropractic has come a long way since Palmer gave his first adjustment in 1895. Today, there are many methods used by chiropractors to correct spinal misalignments, joint dysfunctions and various complexes.

My ultimate goal is to help you improve your body's ability to restore balance and repair itself, which can create remarkable, lasting changes. Chiropractic care offers natural pain relief, allowing you to address the true cause of chronic pain, not just mask the symptoms.

A thorough examination helps locate areas of nervous system compromise. The moving bones of the spine are common culprits. Then, specific chiropractic adjustments help reduce nerve interference. The intent of our work together is to restore your body's ability to regulate and heal itself. Without drugs. Without surgery. Best of all, we have a very high success rate for getting you out of pain and into feeling vital again.

Life is not merely about living, but about living well!

I hope you'll find this information helpful.
Until then, be well!

Brian Kovara, DC

What is Spinal Health?

How many times daily do you stop and think about your spine? If you are like a lot of us, that number sits a solid "zero". As long as we can carry on daily we simply assume everything is just fine, that is unless you suffer from back pain. Those suffering from chronic back pain or back injury have a difficult time getting it off their mind, whether it is the pain itself or coupled with the chain reaction of events that are caused due to it. Back pain is not without cost, monetarily and emotionally.

While most of us do not think of our spinal health on a daily basis, statistics have shown that nearly 80-90% of the population will be affected by spinal issues and back pain at any point during a lifetime. Accident victims aside, those who run the highest risk are smokers, the overweight and heavy lifters. With such a high likelihood there is a solid argument in favor of leading a healthy lifestyle, and in turn, striving for a healthy spine.

Below are some proven strategies for a healthy spine/back:

Healthy Diet and Exercise

Know your ideal body weight and stay within 10 pounds of that weight. Common sense supports the biomechanical logic that carrying around unnecessary body weight will put stress on all areas of the human frame, including the spine.

Strengthen your core muscles. Lack of muscle in this area can pull your entire body out of alignment, starting with your lower back.

Work diligently on eating a reasonably portioned and healthy diet. Couple this diet with a consistent exercise program that fits into your schedule, and you will see results not only in your weight, but in your overall health and confidence.

Always stretch before and after your workout.

Consult with your physician before beginning any diet or exercise program. There may be issues specific to your health conditions that warrant professional guidance.

Smoking Cessation

In terms of physical healing, smokers are far worse off than non-smokers. Blood flow is severely restricted throughout the body by the more-than 4000 chemicals in cigarettes. This restriction slows the healing process to all parts of the body, and the spine is no exception.

Sleeping Habits

Try to support your body as you sleep. Pain at any time is not normal, and if you are feeling pain while you are trying to sleep, find a position that alleviates the pain.

Back sleepers on average place nearly 50 pounds of additional pressure on the spine that can be reduced by nearly half if a supportive pillow is placed under the knees.

Side sleepers can reduce pressure on the spine by placing a pillow between the knees.

Standing

Standing with the knees locked places pressure on the lower back. Relax your stance by placing one foot in front of the other, slightly bending the knees.

Avoid standing bent at the waist for any period of time, this places undue stress on the spine as well.

Lifting

Always engage your legs when lifting. Do not lift solely with your back muscles.

Avoid twisting when lifting anything.

If pushing or pulling an item is an option, choose it. Always choose pushing before pulling, and engage your leg muscles to lessen the strain on the back.

Ask for help.

If carrying the object after lifting, keep it close to the body and spread the weight evenly between both hands.

Sitting

Avoid slumping in your chair. Keep the shoulders back and the spine straight. Do not let your shoulders become rounded or allow your lower back lose its natural curve.

Knees should be slightly higher than the hips.

Keep the head up and looking straight forward.

Bending/Reaching

Bend the legs to pick up items below waist level. Do not bend at the waist.

If reaching for an item higher than shoulder height, use a stool. Straining to reach something above the head can cause injury to the neck, shoulders, and mid-back.

Place your body as close to the object as you reasonably can to further reduce any potential strain.

Like anything in life, there are no guarantees you will avoid back pain, but employing these simple, commonsense strategies certainly increase your chances of leading a pain free, healthy life!

Athletes and Chiropractic Care

Athletes are always looking for an edge to take their performances to another level. No matter what sport you play, the competition is always getting bigger, faster and stronger which means you have to continually improve in order to keep up. Some athletes turn to dishonest methods like performance enhancing drugs to get ahead, but most look to nutrition, enhanced training concepts and similar methods to get better. One way athletes can improve their agility is through chiropractic care.

Enhanced Injury Treatment

Injuries are an unfortunate part of all sports and recovering from injuries quickly and completely is critical. Chiropractic care helps athletes recover from injuries the same way it can help an auto accident victim recover from injuries. Spinal adjustments can align your vertebrae so tendons and muscles heal correctly. If you're experiencing pain from a past injury, chiropractic care can get to the root of the injury and correct the problem, so your symptoms lessen or disappear.

Improved Performance

Athletes can also expect improved overall performance with regular chiropractic care. High-impact athletes can minimize their risk of injury and reduce pain, and low-impact athletes can relieve much of the strain placed on the body while playing their sport. This is true for sports like golf, bowling, and tennis.

With improved strength, balance, stability, flexibility and range of motion, it stands to reason that athletes will notice improved performance with regular chiropractic treatment. For athletes that play through longer seasons or play year-round, the improvement will be noticed as competitors start feeling fatigued and suffering minor injuries. The ability to "stay fresh" from the beginning of the season until the end provides a tremendous advantage to most athletes.

How Chiropractic Helps

Whether it's to enhance performance or help heal an injury, chiropractic helps athletes by taking pressure off nerves in the spinal column. When your spinal vertebrae are misaligned, the impulses sent from your brain to parts of your body through your spine may not be as clear as they should be. When these impulses are restricted, your body is not operating at full capacity, and your athletic performance can suffer. If you are truly looking for an edge and want to take your performance to the next level, try chiropractic treatment and see if it helps. Once the pathways between your brain and muscles, heart and lungs are clear, you'll be amazed at what you can do.

Why Would A Child Benefit from Chiropractic Care?

The spinal cord is the first part of the body to form in the womb, and the nervous system is the "chief controller" of the body.

If its communication channels become damaged, distorted, or fuzzy, the body experiences all sorts of symptoms that may not be obvious they are from the nervous system. While it is important for adults to have chiropractic care, it is equally important for children.

There are so many outside forces that effect an infant right from the start. The baby is compacted into a small space in the mother's womb. Soon after, babies go through significant spinal trauma at birth. Simply from coming out of the birth canal can be taxing on the spine, however other methods of birth can be even more taxing. A C-section birth, vacuum or forceps delivery and induction can be very difficult on a fragile newborn spine.

As infants grow to become toddlers a whole new set of forces are places upon that child. Next as the child learns to walk they are incredibly unsteady on their feet. The average toddler covers more than 2.5 miles per day. This number includes roughly 100 falls. In general, toddlers average about 15 falls per hour. Each fall can reposition their growing spines out of proper alignment.

Additionally, falls, sports injuries, playground bumps, heavy school bags and sitting all day in the classroom are all physical stresses to the growing child's spine and nervous system.

One of the most common reasons for parents to seek chiropractic care for their child is physical trauma from an injury of some sort. The spinal misalignments that may occur at the time of the injury will not necessarily result in immediate pain or symptoms. In addition to physical stress, parents should be aware that emotional and chemical stress affect the child's nervous system and may also warrant a spinal check-up.

Chiropractic Care Helps Children:

* Boost immune system function- lessened number of ear infections

* Promote healthy digestive system- reduced colic and reflux

* Develops nerve resilience

* Improves posture — scoliosis reduction in curvature

* Improves sleep

Regular chiropractic check-ups can identify potential spinal dysfunction resulting from these stresses, and chiropractic adjustments may help to enhance future function and well-being.

It is important to have your children checked as infancy and childhood are impressionable times of rapid growth and development of the spine and nervous system.

Chiropractors examine and evaluate for proper movement, function, and alignment of the spine. Adjustments remove vertebral fixations (joints that are "stuck" and not moving properly) which reduces inflammation and interference to the nervous system. The nervous system controls all of the functions in the entire body. By having your child's spine checked you are maintaining the health of your child's entire body, naturally too! Chiropractic care is gentle and safe. Only light force is needed when adjusting an infant or child's spine. Imagine the pressure needed to press your pinkie-finger into a ripe red tomato and you get the idea.

Chiropractors have the lowest malpractice rates of all primary health care providers in the country, and those rates are based on risk. Actuaries aren't going to give us lower rates without good reason. And as a pediatric chiropractor, my rates are exactly the same as my colleagues who treat adults.".

The key to safety in pediatric chiropractic is education, says Jennifer Brocker, DC, DICCP, who practices with Dr. Hewitt. "It's a completely different process when you work with kids, and you have to know what you're doing in order to treat them appropriately. You need to know the proper techniques, contacts and depth. The contacts need to be smaller and the thrust shallower with less force. Pediatric chiropractic is extremely safe if you know what you're doing, but less so if you don't."

"Children have the same joints that we do, but they're not fully formed yet," adds Emily Watters, DC, who practices in Portland's Whole Mama Whole Child chiropractic and craniosacral clinic. "Their joints are still more cartilaginous than truly bony, so the adjustments have to be a little bit faster but with less force. This is due to the increased flexibility within the joint and the smaller surface area you are targeting. With kids, another option in certain cases is to mobilize joints rather than manipulate them.

"Pediatric chiropractic also differs dramatically from treating adults when it comes to the nature of the complaints. Older children — middle schoolers and teens — may come in with musculoskeletal complaints that resemble those of young adults, particularly if they are involved in athletics. But younger children, toddlers and infants don't usually arrive at the chiropractor's office complaining that they threw their back out after lifting a really heavy Elmo doll or dancing too hard to *The Fresh Beat Band*.

Promotes Healthy Brain and Nerve Development

A baby's nervous system controls everything from breathing, digestion, thinking, sense of touch, and playing. Any damage or disruption can seriously impair his/her ability to function in the best way. Chiropractic helps stimulate a child's brain and nerve activity which creates a balance and a feeling of well-being.

Assists with Asthma, Allergies, and other Breathing Difficulties

When neck muscles become tight, the normal flow of the lymphatic system is interrupted. Since this causes the immune system to become overloaded, chiropractic adjustments help relax neck muscles allowing normal lymphatic drainage. These adjustments help improve the respiratory function which in turn improves symptoms of asthma, allergies, bronchitis, and other breathing problems.

Encourages Good Spinal Posture

Since chiropractic focuses on manipulation of the spine, it helps improve a child's spinal posture. Since the spine is the structure from which the body is built, it is important to begin good postural habits early in life. In addition, birth is very traumatic, and this spinal trauma can lead to many infant issues that can be relieved with simple spinal adjustment by trained Raleigh chiropractors.

Helps with Behavioral Problems

Although chiropractors do not exactly treat behavioral problems in young children, they help eliminate the major stressors of the nervous system. This includes removing spinal subluxations that irritate the nervous system.

Helps with Sleeping Disorders and Bed-wetting Problems

Tension in the neck and back, headaches, joint pain, and other discomforts can prevent proper sleeping patterns. Getting the spine to move properly and in alignment will help relax your child's body to allow better sleep. Chiropractic adjustments also help correct vertebral misalignment (subluxations) which can disturb the proper function of the phrenic reflex and cause bed wetting. Chiropractors correct vertebral subluxations and allow normal function of the phrenic reflex.

Assists with Digestive System

The nervous system controls digestive functions in different regions including lumbar regions, sympathetic nerves that come out of the thoracic, and the sacral parasympathetic nerve fibers. Spinal misalignment in one of these regions may lead to obstructed digestive function. Chiropractic adjustments realign these obstructed regions and help restore nerve supply to the deficient organs.

Helps with Scoliosis

Scoliosis is a condition that involves an abnormal side-to-side curvature of the spine. If not dealt with early in childhood, it is likely to become worse with age. Specific chiropractic adjustments coupled with various muscular rehabilitation techniques can help prevent the progression of scoliosis while the child is still young.

Boosts the Child's Immune System

Chiropractic's purpose is to reduce the interference to a child or baby's nervous system, thus unleashing the full healing power of the body. This helps reduce the occurrence of common colds, ear-aches, and other general illnesses.

It helps with Colic/Irritable Baby Syndrome

Colic or Irritable Baby Syndrome is defined as comfortless crying in a young baby with periodic fussiness that can last for hours. Many babies show improvement with chiropractic care as it involves spinal manipulation to help restore the child's nervous system, digestive tract, and other organs for normal operation.

Promotes Overall Health and Wellbeing

Chiropractic processes make a child healthier, more active and generally happy during growth. . Just as with behavioral problems, the major stressors of the nervous system are eliminated, thus improving your child's concentration in school.

What Does it Mean to Have Disc Trouble?

What are spinal discs? Discs are round and flat on the top and the bottom. They attached securely to the vertebra (spinal bones) both above and below them. There are 23 discs in total which are both flexible and rubbery. The inner core has the consistency of jelly that is made up primarily of water. The discs can be likened to a jelly donut. Shock is absorbed through the discs to allow the spine to bend and twist. As well, discs protect the nerves that run down the middle of the spinal column.

Roughly 1-2% of the population is believed to have a serious bulging disc. More than 50 out of 100 elderly people who undergo an MRI are found to have some degree of a bulging disc. Bulging discs are twice as common in men than in women. The majority of disc bulging occurs in the lower back accounting for 90% of the cases. Only 1% occur within the thoracic spine.

The pain that is felt while having a bulging disc is due to the swelling of the disc, nerve compression and chemical irritation of the nerve.

Overcoming Degenerative Disc Disease

Degenerative disc disease is the deterioration of one or more intervertebral discs of the spine. Degenerative disc usually correlates with the patients age. About 40% of people ages 40 years and up have degenerative disc disease while 80% of 80-year olds will have this disease. The increase in this disease as we age is due to age related weakening. The discs become brittle and dry out which causes the disc to become less flexible and lose its elasticity. Unlike muscles which heal somewhat quickly, degenerative discs heal more slowly.

Living Well Chiropractic & Massage explains that sciatica causes pain and/or numbness/tingling that is brought about by a nerve root irritation that leads to the sciatic nerve. This nerve is the largest single nerve in the whole body. It runs from each side of the spine, through the buttock and into the back side of the thigh down to the foot. Sciatica can be the result of gradual wear and tear over time, old traumas and improper lifting. Symptoms can vary depending on the location. Most occur in the low back causing pain in the buttocks, legs and feet. Nerve irritation in the neck can cause pain in the shoulder, arms and hands. Nerve roots act as a telegraph line to other parts of the body and can cause pain felt in other parts of the body. The radiating pain that is felt is referred to as radiculopathy.

Disc issues are generally diagnosed through a thorough history and physical. Your chiropractor at Living Well Chiropractic & Massage will check your range of motion and pain level. X-rays are usually the first step in imaging with a possible MRI. After the data has all been collected and a diagnosis has been established, your chiropractor will decide on the best treatment plan for you.

Early into an acute episode, a chiropractor will set a goal of pain control by using several modalities within the office. Spinal manipulation will help to realign the spinal bones while exercise will be helpful to strengthen the surrounding muscles to support your spine.

Decompression is widely used as a non-surgical and pain free method to help create additional space between the discs and relieve symptoms of numbness/tingling and radiculopathy. The spine is gently stretched and relaxed intermittently in a controlled manner to help pull back the bulging material back into the disc while also promoting the passage of nutrients into the disc for a more efficient healing environment.

How to Avoid Back Injury

When it comes to avoiding back injuries, your fate is largely in your own hands. It's true that an unexpected fall or auto accident may cause an injury that's beyond your control, but a large percentage of back injuries are caused by your own actions, which means you can take measures to prevent them or stop them from getting worse. Here are a few valuable back injury avoidance techniques:

Pay Attention to Your Lifting Technique

How you lift boxes, laundry baskets, children's toys, a pair of shoes or just about anything else, has a bearing on the health of your back. When you lift correctly your spine is in the proper alignment and there is no added stress placed on your back. This means you should bend your knees and keep your back as straight as possible when you pick anything up off the floor.

If you have a lot of lifting to do, try to place items on a table or chair so there isn't as much bending required picking it up. Your back is not designed to work like a crane so anytime you use it that way you are putting stress on your back that doesn't need to be there. Take a balanced stance, lift with your legs and move your feet if you need to change direction while holding the object.

Sensible Body Management

Performing activities with your back health in mind is a great strategy to help you avoid back injuries. That means stretching before any type of physical activity, taking it slow if you have a lot of repetitive lifting to do, and taking breaks to rest and stretch during the activity.

Getting yourself into good physical condition also protects your back and helps to avoid injuries. This includes losing weight in your midsection, and strengthening core muscles, to make lifting and general movement less stressful on your back. Most chiropractors will tell you that sleeping on a firm mattress is another way you can nurture your back and prevent injuries.

Don't Let Injuries Linger

If you end up with a back injury despite your efforts to avoid it, you should seek treatment with a chiropractor as soon as you can. Spinal misalignment, bulging discs, herniated discs, and other injuries often only get worse if you let them linger. Prompt treatment will restore blood flow to the area, relieve any compressed nerves and get you back to normal in the shortest time possible.

Three Tips to Keep Your Body Running Smoothly

Since chiropractors see the results of poor lifestyle choices on a daily basis, it's only natural to formulate opinions and offer tips to patients so they can help themselves. From sore backs, necks, shoulders, irregular sleeping patterns to back pain, we provide help in a wide range of areas.

Here are three tips that will help keep your body operating efficiently.

1) Try Not to Sit So Much

Sitting seems like a relatively innocent activity, but the negative effects that prolonged sitting creates are numerous. Extensive sitting has always been associated with back pain and spinal issues, but recent research also suggests a link between too much sitting and heart disease. If you have a sedentary job like so many people do, make a point of getting up and moving around at least once per hour. You can take phone calls standing up, buy an adjustable standing desk, do deep knee bends, jumping jacks or just go for a quick walk. The key is to stand up and move around to relieve pressure and stay healthy.

2) Get Injuries Treated Promptly

Another important tip from a chiropractic team is to get quick treatment if you've suffered an injury. A little twist or tweak now can lead to years of discomfort and improper muscle function if you just leave it alone. It's always wise to apply ice to injuries to help reduce swelling but visiting a chiropractor as soon as possible will help with the healing process and keep your muscles and joints functioning at full capacity.

Leaving minor injuries may not cause a great deal of pain, but the effects will be felt in the future. Many people end up using various pain medications or having reduced mobility as they get older because they chose to leave an injury alone.

3) Incorporate Stretching Into Your Day

Treating injuries promptly is a good idea but preventing them altogether is even better. Keeping your muscles, tendons, and ligaments flexible with daily stretching will help you avoid many common injuries. You can incorporate the stretches into your morning routine or as part of your daily workout regimen. As you age, those muscles will become tighter and tighter leaving you prone to injury. Working for long hours hunched over a desk also shortens muscles and opens the door to injury. Stretching tips from a chiropractor include your hamstrings, quadriceps, calves, chest, hips, and back. It only takes a few minutes a day, but you'll notice the results for the rest of your life.

Five Tips for Dealing with Back Pain

Our patients have always appreciated our 5 Tips for Back Pain. Have you missed work, had to give up a recreational activity that you enjoy, or had trouble sleeping at night because of back pain? If so you're not alone. In fact, it was recently found that 80% of Americans will experience back pain at some point throughout their lives. In addition to this startling statistic, back pain has also risen to capture the number one spot as the leading cause of disability in the United States. While pain is the primary concern for sufferers of back pain, it often causes a significant financial burden as well. In 2012 alone, it was estimated that the American people spent nearly 30 billion dollars seeking treatment for their back pain.

With back pain rising to epidemic proportions, patients, doctors, and researchers are searching high and low for a cost-effective solution. Our team at

Living Well Chiropractic & Massage hopes this article will give you some information on the latest discoveries in research about back pain.

Five Simple Tips to Help You Manage Your Back Pain:

1. While being overweight or obese has been shown to be correlated with a greater incidence of heart attack, stroke, and diabetes, it has also been found to be one of the biggest contributing factors for the development of back pain. Since our body's frame is designed to only carry a certain amount of weight, excess weight puts an immense strain not only on our spine, but also on other joints throughout our body. This excess strain has been shown to increase the rate of degeneration of the vertebrae in our back, leading to the early development of back pain.

In addition to the degenerative effects of being overweight, those extra pounds have been shown to increase the odds of developing osteoarthritis, a herniated disc, and sciatica. Unfortunately, people who are obese also have a greater tendency to undergo unwanted back surgeries. So, the next time you feel the urge to stop at your favorite fast food establishment, think twice and head home to get some of those fresh fruits and veggies.

2. Since the time that cigarettes were invented there has always been someone saying smoking is bad for you. While many people have heard that smoking increases the risk of cancer, these same people may be surprised to hear that research is showing it also contributes to the development of back pain. In fact, smoking is related to spinal pain in a couple of different ways. First of all, smoking has been identified as one of the main factors in causing atherosclerosis (blockage of the small arteries throughout the body). The spine and its related tissues such, as the intervertebral discs, primarily receive their blood supply and nutrients from these small vessels. As these structures become obstructed due to

smoking, the tissues are unable heal properly leading to early degeneration and pain.

In addition to the effects of atherosclerosis, the nicotine that is found in cigarettes has been shown to decrease the activity of the bone forming cells called osteoblasts. This can be considered another contributing factor to the spines decreased healing capability and as a direct result the presence of pain. These findings only give you another reason to quit smoking.

3. I bet you can still remember your parents yelling at you to sit up straight while at the dinner table or doing your homework. While you may have rebelled against your parents then, you should listen now; your posture has a large effect on your spine and the development of back pain. With the increased time people spend in the seated position at work or on the computer at home, learning how to correct your posture will go a long way in helping you obtain relief from back pain.

The effects of poor posture range from putting extra strain on the discs, vertebrae, and muscles throughout your back to causing an increase in pressure on the nerves exiting the spine. All of these factors contribute to pain not only in your back, but also throughout other areas of your body. So, the next time you think about slouching in your chair, sit up straight and follow your chiropractor's advice.

4. Have you ever noticed that you back pain becomes worse when sitting in one position for too long? It has been shown through research that inactivity is one of the primary factors for the development of long-term musculoskeletal pain. Not only does inactivity lead to weight gain (which causes back pain in itself), it also causes the structures that support the spine to weaken, resulting in a greater incidence of back pain. In addition to weakening, the muscles and discs tend to shorten as certain positions are maintained for long periods of time. Simply developing a daily exercise

and stretching program can go a long way in helping you gain relief from your back pain.

5. While many people wait until they can hardly stand the pain to visit a chiropractor, it is important to understand that pain is your body's last mechanism for letting you know something is wrong. While the effectiveness and safety of chiropractic for the treatment of lower back pain is undebatable, many people are still unaware of exactly how chiropractic helps.

Chiropractors simply focus on allowing the body to function properly, typically concentrating on the musculoskeletal and nervous system. While each patient is treated individually depending on their condition, chiropractors are skilled at identifying and correcting spinal misalignments. Since every message from your brain to your body travels through your spinal cord you can imagine how important the alignment of your spinal bones is for protecting this important structure. While chiropractic has been shown to be one of the most cost-effective treatments for back pain, chiropractors are even better at preventing back pain from beginning in the first place.

How Do Massage and Chiropractic Care Work Together?

Massage therapy dates back thousands of years. In the 1850's two American doctors who were studying in Sweden brought massage therapy to the United States. Today, it has been said that roughly 50 million adult Americans had a massage at least one time in the past year. Fifty percent of those sought out massage for a medical or health reason while 28 percent were seeking relaxation massage.

Different Types of Massage Offered

There are several different types of massage at Living Well aimed to suit each individual patient's needs.

- Swedish (the most popular)
- Deep Tissue
- Hot Stone

- Shiatsu

- Pregnancy

- Reflexology

- Sports

- Thai

Benefits of Massage Therapy

- Pain reduction – headaches, sports injuries, chronic pain

- Relaxation

- Increased circulation

- Immune function booster

- Reducing scar tissue

- Increased range of motion

- Lower blood pressure

- Lymphatic drainage

Massage may also help to reduce digestive problems as the increased circulation aids in relaxing the lower back and abdominal muscles.

With therapeutic massage, patients tend to feel improvement, however one massage will typically not resolve a lifelong history with chronic pain. There is a cumulative effect. It took years to create the imbalance, pain and structural changes and it will take time to fix it as well. Often times, home exercises are given in between appointments to help improve results.

Massage is an excellent modality when used in conjunction with chiropractic. Patients find themselves healing and recovering faster when both the muscular and skeletal issues are addressed simultaneously. Together, the two disciplines restore mobility and functionality.

Three Common Conditions Chiropractors Address

Chiropractic is a treatment method that has moved from more of an alternative treatment to widespread mainstream acceptance over the past few decades. There will always be pockets of naysayers that question its validity, but the millions of satisfied patients around the world speak volumes about the effectiveness of chiropractic treatment on the human body. There are literally dozens of health issues that benefit from chiropractic adjustments, but here are 3 common conditions that chiropractors help:

1) Headaches — We all get headaches from time to time. Some are mild, some are more severe, but all of them have the potential to disrupt your day. Whether it is a tension headache caused by hours of sitting at a desk or a migraine brought on by a specific health condition, when the pain starts it is difficult to focus on anything else.

Chiropractors help relieve headache pain on a regular basis. A lot of the time the pain you feel in your head is actually being caused by misalignment of the vertebrae in your spine. After a gentle adjustment and proper maintenance, many patients report no more pain and no more need for pain medication.

2) Shoulder Pain — Shoulder pain is a problem that far too many people deal with. Pain in the shoulder can be referred pain from the spinal misalignments, or it can be caused by a misalignment in the shoulder.

No matter what specific type of shoulder pain you have, chiropractors help relieve both the pain and any range of motion issues that are present. Our team will help to access your condition and give you the best advice we can on what you can do to remedy the situation.

3) Lower Back Pain — If headaches and shoulder pain are among the most common conditions for the general public then lower back pain is probably at the head of the pack. One of the most common reasons for lumbar pain is from misaligned spinal segments.

Our team can help the pain and reduced mobility associated with lumbar strains and sprains and help patients get back to their normal routines. Even if you've had lower back pain for years and have been told there is nothing that will help, it's always worth the time explore your possibilities.

How Long Do Patients See Chiropractors?

One belief that many people pick up is that once you begin chiropractic treatment for a specific health issue you must continue with that treatment forever. Anyone that has visited a chiropractor knows that the patient is always in control and any recommendations regarding treatment length aren't set in stone.

How Long Do I Need Chiropractic Care?

In reality, there is no concrete answer to the question of how long you need chiropractic care because every situation is different. If patient A tweaked her lower back picking up a basket of laundry and patient B injured several cervical vertebrae in a car accident, the treatment plans and lengths will be quite different.

The only way to really know for sure is to book a consultation with a chiropractor and start your treatment. It's not uncommon for different people to respond differently to the same treatments, so even if two people have the same issue the treatment length can vary. Most of the time chiropractors will recommend regular treatments until the patient is no longer symptomatic, then it's up to you if you want to continue.

The length of time it takes to eliminate your back pain, headaches, neck pain, shoulder pain, or whatever is ailing you depends on the severity of the problem and your own physical make up. If you are in good physical condition and take care of yourself, you'll probably heal faster than someone who doesn't.

Patients Always Maintain Control

Even if you decide that you want to discontinue treatment before your symptoms have completely gone, no one is going to try and force you to stay. You may be given a breakdown of what is likely to happen and why it is important for your healing to continue, but no reputable chiropractor would try to make a patient do something they don't want to do. This is part of the reason why most chiropractors are so forthcoming with information at the beginning of the process.

Benefits of Long-Term Maintenance

It's important to note that many patients will opt for periodic maintenance even after chiropractors have relieved their initial symptoms. It's not unusual to see patients coming into the office that have no pain or discomfort at all. This is how you keep those underlying issues from popping up again and causing trouble like they did the first time. A long-term preventative treatment plan is usually advised after you're healed, but this is also completely the patient's decision.

Sciatica is Literally a Pain in the Butt!

Got Pain? — here take this pain pill. That's what the big pharmaceutical companies want you to do. However, more and more people are bucking the system. They are tired of sticking on a Band-Aid in the form a drug. They realize the harm that taking pain medications long term can have on their bodies. They also understand that they are not having the symptom due to a "lack of Vicodin" in their body. Are you sick and tired of popping pills and looking for answers to the root cause so you can effectively treat the problem and not merely mask the symptoms? If so, read on.

The truth is that many people do or will suffer with sciatica. It is estimated that approximately 40% of the population will experience sciatica at some point in their life. Sciatica refers to pain due to irritation to the sciatic nerve. It can be exceptionally painful and quite debilitating. The sciatic nerve is the largest nerve in the human body and runs from the lower spine to the bottom of the foot. When irritated, the sciatic nerve can elicit pain anywhere along the nerve's pathway.

The most common cause of sciatica is when the spinal nerve roots from the lumbosacral (lower back) region become pinched due to spinal misalignments (subluxations) or from an intervertebral disk bulge or herniation. Other potential causes could be due to muscle spasms in the lower back, hip or pelvis. Each of these causes are mechanical problems that create physical stress to the sciatic nerve. Since they are physical in nature, they would obviously require a physical solution to the problem. That is why chemical treatments (pain relieving drugs) don't fix the underlying cause but merely block the pain signal to the brain. This is where differential diagnosis becomes so important. Once you determine the underlying cause and location, a specific treatment plan can be created.

Treatment of sciatica varies in length with most people returning to normal activities within 6 weeks. At my clinic on Bainbridge Island, I treat sciatica, from an origin of spinal and disk issues, with a course of spinal adjustments and/or spinal decompression therapy. I also utilize natural supplements to reduce inflammation and pain. For muscular involvement, massage therapy is often included in treatment planning. I also focus on exercise training to strengthen and stabilize core muscles to avoid future episodes.

Has Plantar Fasciitis got you off on the wrong foot?

New solutions to naturally resolve the pesky foot pain.

Plantar fasciitis is a common problem I see in the office. More and more people are coming in with complaints of sharp, stabbing and burning pain in the bottom of their feet especially after sleeping or sitting for a while. If you are reading this, does it sound familiar?

Let me start by explaining what fascia is. Fascia is a thin layer of tissue that lays over muscles. The sole of your foot is also called the plantar surface. Hence the name plantar fascia. So, what is fasciitis? Itis means inflammation, so fasciitis is inflammation of fascia. Now the foot itself acts much like a tripod with the three points being the heel, in addition to points on the medial (inner part) and lateral (outer part) of the ball of the foot. These three points create the three arches of the foot: the medial (inner), lateral (outer) and transverse (across) arches. If the bones of the foot move out of place, they affect the integrity of the three arches, and cause stress to the plantar fascia. So plantar fasciitis is an inflammation of the soft tissue on the bottom of the foot that can be brought on by macro or micro traumas. Macro trauma could be from jumping or falling from a large elevation, and micro trauma is more of a repetitive stress type injury.

My experience is that the vast majority of cases are from the micro trauma variety. So, what causes repetitive stress to your feet? Walking or running for long distances. It can also be from years of being on your feet if you work or worked at a job that required lots of standing or walking. When we stand or walk, the tissues in the bottom of the foot undergo a large amount of strain from carrying our body weight. The more overweight we are, the more the stress to the feet. This stress creates a ripping of the fascia. When you are off your feet, the tissue shortens, then gets re-torn if when you stand up again.

Repairing of the plantar fasciitis requires a multifaceted approach. We need to address the joints of the feet, stabilize and support the arches and treat the soft tissue injury. Adjustments to the bones of the feet, taping of the arches and/or orthotics will help to support the arches and treatment of the soft tissue could include massage, rapid release therapy, laser treatment, and more.

Sitting is the New Smoking

As modern technology continues to evolve it seems that people are sitting more and more. With smart phones and tablets such a big part of everyday life many of the activities that used to be physical are now played out without having to move much at all. It's not uncommon for someone to get out of bed, sit in a car on the way to work, sit all day at a desk, sit in the car on the way home, and then sit all evening watching television or playing with their smart phone.

The Trouble with Sitting

Many people will look at the previous paragraph and say they have no choice but to commute to work and sit at a desk. This may be true, but excessive sitting is rough on your back and it's also bad for your overall health. Many visits to a chiropractor deal with back pain and related back issues, and too much sitting is one of the main culprits. Even if your chair feels comfortable and has been deemed "ergonomically sound", it is still a bad idea to maintain a prolonged static posture. Even the most advanced office chairs can't reverse the force of gravity.

Aside from back pain, prolonged sitting will flatten out your butt and tighten up your hips and hamstrings, leaving you prone to injury when you exercise. Sitting too much also promotes more serious health concerns such as increased risk of blood clots, increased risk of heart disease, type 2 diabetes, and weight gain. Research has shown that these health risks aren't improved with one workout per day if you sit for too long. You have to take matters into your own hands and start moving more.

What to Do If You Have a Sedentary Job

The reason sitting too much is dangerous for your spine is because when you sit you're putting almost twice the stress on your spine as you would if you were standing. If you're the type to hunch forward slightly in your chair, the problem gets even worse. When you have your shoulders forward your back makes "C" shape removing the natural curve at the bottom of the spine.

If you are among the many thousands with sedentary jobs, you can make a few tweaks to your routine to protect your back and ward off the more serious ailments associated with too much sitting. First, try your best not to slouch forward. Sit up straight with your shoulders back and maintain your natural arch in the low back.

Next, make yourself get up and out of your chair at least once every 30 minutes. Take a walk around the office, do some light stretches or just stand, but make sure you get up. If you have access to a standing desk use it for a portion of each day. The key is to take short movement breaks every day, so your muscles, tendons, and ligaments stay loose and flexible. If you have a sore back from too much sitting, a visit to your chiropractor will help get things back in balance and remove your pain.

How Do We Boost Our Immune System?

Everyone knows that your ability to ward off disease and remain healthy has a lot to do with your immune system. Through the years we've been taught and programmed to believe a shot or prescription medication will give us the immune system support we need, but this isn't always true. In fact, some of the keys to a healthy immune system are situated in your joints and vertebrae right now, and chiropractors have the tools to give your immunity a boost.

Misalignment and Your Immune System

It is crucial that your brain and nervous system communicate clearly with each other for an effective immune response. If your nervous system is not functioning at full capacity, then your immune system may not be working with 100% effectiveness. This means greater susceptibility to viruses, bacteria, and disease. When you have misaligned vertebrae, known as subluxations, the corresponding nerves can be affected making the communication with your brain muddled and possibly decreasing the immune response.

How Chiropractic Adjustment Boosts Immunity

Chiropractic adjustments can remove misalignments, allowing the nerves in your spine to operate with less interference. When the brain and nervous system are able to communicate effectively your immune system is back running at full capacity. Chiropractic doctors may also reduce your back pain, neck pain, jaw pain, headaches, and shoulder pain so you can function in your day-to-day life more efficiently. While chiropractic treatment can influence your immune system directly, it can also heal your body, so you are in a position to be more active.

Immune Support and Children

Kids seem to be at the mercy of just about every type of virus and illness out there and childhood immunity is always a hot topic of conversation. Things like ear infections, colds, allergies, and tonsillitis can cause a lot of discomfort and become serious in some cases. Just as with adults, children can receive chiropractic treatment that will ease tension on nerves and improve their immune response.

With problems like ear infections, chiropractic adjustment can help to drain the Eustachian tube in the inner ear which becomes plugged and is responsible for the formation of bacteria and viruses. Our chiropractors at Living Well Chiropractic & Massage are well versed at performing spinal adjustments on children and most parents notice a reduction in cold or flu symptoms after a visit. As long as the immune system remains strong the body is more protected. Chiropractic care can make a real difference for your family.

Why Take Health Advice from a Chiropractor?

The saying, "If you don't have your health, you have nothing" is true for every person of every age in every country on earth. It's easy to get side-tracked into believing work or your relationships are the most important things, but when a serious health issue creeps in, you quickly realize that nothing else matters. Even something relatively minor like a misaligned disc in your cervical spine can cause headaches that will have you on your back in a darkened room. Here is some valuable health advice from a chiropractor that will help you to live a pain-free, disease-free life.

Take a Whole-Body Approach

Many people believe true health is something that can be had by visiting the gym a few times per week and downing some supplements before each meal. Being healthy in a whole-body sense includes several other factors that should all be working in unison with the physical part. These include your emotional health, social health, occupational health, intellectual health, and your relationship with the environment.

This may sound like a lot of factors, but they are all important. If they weren't, every top athlete would be completely content and living a life that makes them happy daily because they are physically healthy. Obviously, this is not the case and it is because some of the other health elements are not being met. Being free from emotional traumas, anxiety and depression, loving what you do every day, and having a strong social network to share your life with all help create a healthy person.

Move Your Body Everyday

Movement is one of the key factors to keeping your body strong and flexible. It can also help to release chemicals in your brain that make you feel good. You don't have to go to the gym and you don't have to play an organized sport, but you should engage in some sort of physical activity every day. An exercise plan or recommendation is part of any health advice you'd receive from a chiropractors.

The Role of Chiropractic

For most people the road to total health isn't starting with a perfectly clean slate. You've already suffered injuries or had health issues that require some attention. When you visit our chiropractic team, you'll be assessed and a treatment plan will be created that will likely include chiropractic adjustments and other techniques. Relieving tension in your joints and spinal column can provide tremendous benefits by eliminating pain and allowing blood to flow freely. Chiropractic treatment is a valuable first step on the road to a healthy life.

Doctors of the Future According to Thomas Edison

Doctors of the future will give no medicine but will interest their patients in the care of the human frame, in diet and in the cause and prevention of disease.
~ Thomas Edison

What does it mean to be physically healthy?

Physical wellness is something most of us aspire to; very few of us (over 40) is without complaint in terms of our mobility and sense of balance. When we are physically healthy, we usually feel happy in spirit and in our bodies. How do we measure physical health?

In ancient times — both Eastern and Western — the gauge of wellness was a sense of mind-body balance. Even in the 21st-century, the Centers for Disease Control and Prevention (CDCP) write, "Health is a state of complete physical, mental, and social well-being, and not merely the absence of disease or infirmity."

The CDC has a questionnaire entitled "Healthy Days Measures" and the questions they include are the following:

- Would you say that in general your health is excellent, very good, good, fair or poor?

- Now thinking about your physical health, which includes physical illness and injury, how many days during the past 30 days was your physical health not good?

- Now thinking about your mental health, which includes stress, depression, and problems with emotions, how many days during the past 30 days was your mental health not good?

- During the past 30 days, approximately how many days did poor physical or mental health keep you from doing your usual activities, such as self-care, work, or recreation?

How do we know we are healthy?

One of the ways we think about our health is when it is missing. For instance, when we feel physical stress, we often have physical symptoms arise. Physical stress can be born of or even lead to poor nutrition, poor sleep, and physical injury.

Our bodies release adrenaline when we are stressed to help us have quick energy to cope. Whether the stress is physical danger, like being chased by a gorilla, or emotional, such as a break-up, death of a loved one or job loss, the physical effects of adrenaline in the body (especially for long periods) is wearing. Given all this, it is easy to see how stress causes excessive wear and damage that leaves us exhausted. Such burnout leads us to reaching for artificial substances alcohol or drugs to relax or caffeine to give us a boost to keep going. By adding these chemicals, we've just doubled the amount of manageable stress.

For example: when we're in a panic we become saturated with stress hormones like adrenaline, cortisol and norepinephrine. This saturation results in a "shut down" response; a pattern that creates not only sleep deprivation and exhaustion but a sluggish metabolism. Experts agree, when you're not balanced, you are more likely to shovel in quick energy, chemically-manufactured, high-sugar foods and skip workouts. When amped up or exhausted (same hormonal coin), who wants to eat whole foods, move more intentionally, or even workout?

Motion is life!

In chiropractic school, we learn that the human body is a complex system of bones, joints, muscles, and nerves, designed to work together to accomplish one thing: motion. Even the ancient founders of the Olympic games, (in honor of the god Zeus), 2700 years ago held the slogan "motion is life."

As a matter of fact, research has shown that motion is so critical to our health that a lack of motion has a detrimental effect on everything from digestion to our emotional state, immune function, our ability to concentrate, how well we sleep and even to how long we live. If our lifestyle does not include enough motion, our body cannot function efficiently.

According to Dr. Richard Andreasen, there are three ways we know we are unhealthy: "First, you will not be as physically healthy and will suffer from a wide variety of physical ailments, ranging from headaches to high blood pressure. Second, you will not be as productive in your life because of reduced energy levels and the lack of ability to mentally focus. Third, because you have less energy, your activity level will tend to drop off even further over time, creating a downward spiral of reduced energy and less activity until you get to a point where even the demands of a sedentary job leave you physically exhausted at the end of the day."

Why must we have good posture?

Chiropractors believe that the human body craves alignment and claim when properly aligned, our bones, not simple our muscles, support our weight, reducing effort and strain. The big payoff with proper posture is that we feel healthier, have more energy, and move gracefully. So, while the word "posture" may conjure up images of book-balancing charm-school girls, it is not just about standing up straight. It is about being aware of and connected to every part of yourself.

Maintaining mobility is critical in order to live free from pain and disability. Maintaining good mobility is not difficult for most of us, but it does not happen on its own. Just as in developing a good posture, it is necessary that you perform specific exercises and stretches to keep muscles, ligaments, and tendons flexible and healthy. In addition, it is necessary that all of the joints in our body are kept moving correctly as well. Although this can be achieved to a great degree through stretching, most people also find routine chiropractic adjustments to be very beneficial.

Questions for Reflection:

- How do I take care of myself physically?

- How do I know when I'm out of balance physically?

- What small action am I willing to take to improve my physical range of motion?

- How will I celebrate progress in physical self-care?

What Helps Carpal Tunnel Syndrome?

Carpal Tunnel Syndrome is a medical condition that affects many people. It is often a work-related injury affecting adults that perform repetitive tasks with their hands. This includes people that work on computers for long periods of time and assembly line workers in various industries. Carpal Tunnel Syndrome (CTS) is a common injury that a chiropractor treats, especially when conventional medicine has failed to provide help.

What Is Carpal Tunnel Syndrome?

Carpal Tunnel Syndrome refers to compression of the median nerve that runs from your forearm into your hand. The nerve gets compressed in a narrow tunnel in your wrist, known as the carpal tunnel. This tunnel consists of soft tissues, bones, tendons, nerves, ligaments, and blood vessels.

Symptoms of CTS

When you have CTS, common symptoms include pain and weakness in the hand and wrist area that often results in numbness or tingling radiating up to the forearm. More specifically, the palm of your hand, thumb, middle fingers, and index fingers feel the bulk of the discomfort. Many CTS sufferers feel as though their hands and fingers are swollen and puffy, even though no swelling is evident. Without proper treatment from a chiropractor, Carpal Tunnel Syndrome can make it difficult to form a fist, affect grip strength, and cause muscle wasting at the base of the thumb. Some CTS sufferers lose sensation in their hands and are no longer able to distinguish between hot and cold.

Diagnosing CTS

Some people have a higher likelihood of developing Carpal Tunnel Syndrome because they have smaller carpal tunnels in their wrists than others. Smaller tunnels increase the likelihood of nerve compression increasing the risk of CTS. When diagnosing CTS your chiropractor will give you a physical examination to see if your symptoms fall in line with the injury. You'll be asked to perform some rudimentary wrist exercises and they may try some specific pressure and compression tests to test the sensitivity of the nerve. You might also be required to have an x-ray or other imaging tests to rule out other wrist injuries or conditions.

Getting Treatment

Once the CTS diagnosis has been established you'll have to rest the affected hand and wrist and possibly immobilize your wrist to prevent further damage. Applying ice to the area to reduce swelling may also be part of the treatment, depending on the severity of the condition. Joint adjustments and light stretching and strengthening exercises will likely be part of your chiropractic treatment. Chiropractors often find that the spine is also involved in causing this symptom.

Each treatment is customized to suit the individual and with regular sessions your CTS pain and other symptoms should subside.

When the Weather Outside is Frightful: Ten Ways of Staying Active Indoors

1. Have a dance party — crank up the funky music and get moving. Move the furniture around so you have a large open space. March, stomp, twirl, jump, and hop. If it appeals to you, get out some fun musical instruments. Get your friends, colleagues or family members to join in and have fun!

2. Hit the gym with a Buddy — do jumping jacks, burpees, yoga, Pilates, Zumba or push ups, try sit ups, jump rope or even run in place. If you have experience, do some strength training.

3. Get indoor basketball hoops — if you have the space and don't mind playing with balls inside. This is an awesome way to kick it with adults or kids.

4. Go up and down the stairs — Kids and other energizer bunnies love to climb up and down the stairs! If you can keep it up for 20 minutes, you've jogged two miles.

5. Get an indoor trampoline – You can torch 160 calories in half an hour of jumping on your mini-trampoline, and it's low-impact, too. "You get an amazing workout and it's so much fun," says Basheerah Ahmad, founder of the fitness consulting firm 360 Transformation.

6. Play any sport, even dance, with interactive video games – Wii Fit is aimed at everyone, says Nintendo. The company created the video exercise game to go with its original Wii console, which boasts virtual games of tennis, bowling, baseball, boxing, and golf. You need to own that Wii – or buy one, for about $250 – to be able to use it, of course. For an additional $90, you get a CD full of exercises, information, and the all-important balance board.

7. Create an indoor "ice rink" – polish the floor with Mr. Sheen or another similar product and let the kids go "ice skating" using socks as their skates. Be sure they don't get too rough or careless with this one or you'll be dealing with injuries or broken furniture.

8. Play active games like Twister or Charades as opposed to board games that keep you sitting.

9. Visit a local indoor pool — it is low cost to belong to the local YMCA. A family membership is very inexpensive and gives you privilege to so much, including a wonderful indoor pool facility. If you do not have a YMCA in your area you may want to check out another local fitness center. Call and ask for a tour. Inquire about a free two-week trial.

10. Go bowling — Bowling helps promote muscle exercise of the lower body, as you are doing a lot of walking with the extra weight of a bowling ball in your hands. Further, when you are swinging your arm to throw the bowling ball, the stretching and flexing that occurs provides enough exercise for the tendons, ligaments, muscles and joints in your arms. The trick is to learn how to bowl correctly otherwise injury is inevitable.

What ways do you stay fit indoors? We would love to add to this list!

So Long Summer: Making Seasonal Transitions Without Losing Ground

Adios Summer

Saying goodbye to the longer days of summer will not be easy for those of us who wait all year for the sunny season — especially those of us from the "rust belt" here in the PNW. However, the last few weeks before fall can be a time to hit the reset button in terms of our health and wellness practices.

To help you transition more smoothly from the summer season, here are some supportive methods to get into the fall groove.

You Can't Make Me Say Goodbye

Saying goodbye to people or things can bring out the blues in anyone (even our pets). Think about what helps you when a vacation is over. I call this "re-entry" and notice I often need to take time to re-organize myself and my stuff. I don't need to do a thorough spring cleaning but do need to consider a new routine if I'm going to keep up (or even begin) a program of health and wellness when the weather cools, I'm going to need some mental time to strategize for success.

What If I Feel Out of Balance?

Making a list of my aspirations for a balanced season may include exercise, sleep, proper nutrition, setting new goals, scheduling down time, beginning (or getting back into) a meditation practice, organizing social gatherings, making time for fun and leisure, and/or even establishing a new hobby. Learning to stay energized and rested is vital if I'm going to feel healthy all fall. Remembering what has worked in past autumns can be a great way to uncover what can support me in the present.

How Will I Find and Eat Fresh Foods?

Again, making a list of what's growing locally can be easier if you head to the local Farmer's Market. If you don't have one, try shopping the outer perimeter of your grocery store; that's where all the whole/fresh foods are kept. The closer you move to the center, ironically, the more likely you'll find "foods" that aren't really food but a *mish mash* of chemicals, starch, salt and sugar-laden ingredients that have been aging for quite a while.

As I've said in another blogpost, let's follow scientist Michael Pollan's advice: "Eat food, not too much, mostly plants." Probably the first two words are most important. "Eat food" means to eat real food — vegetables, fruits, whole grains, and, yes, fish and meat — and avoid what Pollan calls "edible food-like substances," those manufactured "foods" you have to unwrap from their packages.

NOTE: *If it doesn't rot within a week or your great grandmother couldn't find it in her home, it is toxic no matter how many times the word natural is written on its packaging.*

Planning ahead for meals also supports you and the entire family (if that applies). Be sure to shop for the week then pick one or two days to prep your snacks and meals for school or work in advance. Pack smaller containers with seeds, nuts, fresh-cut veggies, and fruits to stay healthy on the go. The key is to get creative, keep it simple and delicious, while keeping it healthy.

What about Flu Season?

The flu is not so much about germs but the result of a combination of things that stop your body from adapting to the environment, mainly because of the CHANGE in seasons.

- Decreased activity levels because we are inside more

- Decreased water consumption because of the decrease in temperature and activity

- Decreased vitamin D because of less sunlight exposure

- Increased sugar consumption is all too common with cold weather

- Increased stress levels

Prevention is the goal and being mindful to what supports us is a beginning.

How Do I Stay Fit?

Whether your 10 or 100, moving every day for at least 30-minutes will help you feel good and avoid the downside to the season — colds, weight gain, exhaustion, stress, blues and sleep problems.

Whether you're hitting the gym, taking a yoga class, cycling, or swimming, choose an activity that you will challenge you AND be one you enjoy. Why? Because if it's fun, you'll keep doing it!

Accountability helps, so grab a friend to keep yourself growing.

Where Does Chiropractic Care Come In?

Your chiropractor can guide you to define what is balance for you? Check with her or him before starting any new fitness regime and learn ways to prevent physical problems that can arise with your new program. Being aware of any past injuries or health problems ahead of time — such as heart disease, diabetes, or arthritis — will make all the difference in the world.

While chiropractic care won't fix everything, i.e., set a broken bone, they do know how to keep you aligned with the natural healing flow of your nervous system; it's the basement of our house. Without a firm foundation, our progress will be set in sand — no more secure than the sandcastles we see disappear at the end of a summer day.

What Will Massage Do for Me?

Massage affects our entire circulatory system to flush out toxins and carry immune cells throughout the body to help defend against infections. As our massage therapist Brigette Milne says, "It's all about the lymph system." If our lymph fluid circulation gets sluggish, toxins can accumulate, and immune cells may not get carried to the areas of the body where they are needed most.

Unlike our heart, our lymph system doesn't have a pump for circulation. And lack of flow, (beyond gravity), we will leave us feeling out-of-balance: more aches, constipation, pains and swelling (lymph edema).

Therapeutic Massage can work like our own heart to be a strong pump that gives us what we need and releases what doesn't serve us.

When There is No Time, Make Time

The modern world has trained us to be distraction-consumption oriented. Whether we are running errands or checking social media, we lose our focus when we are trapped in a frenzy of accomplishing and acquiring. We spend the majority of our days plugged in to something that is outwardly focused whether it's our "smartphones" or our unruly to do list. Unless we're able to balance our lives with down time, we may find ourselves overloaded or exhausted.

Medical doctor and spiritual guru Deepak Chopra considers down time to be "doing no mental work and just letting the mind and brain simply be." Taking a hot bath, gazing at a fire in the hearth, meditating, or listening to music can be incredibly nourishing down-time fall activities.

Unplugging from too-much stimulation allows us to rest and reboot, which gives us the focus and stamina to take on work or other challenges.

A Few Simple Things to Remember...

A smooth transition from summer to fall comes down to identifying how we want to spend our time and creating healthy new habits. A small shift in perspective and a bit of paying attention to our priorities will help get us into the groove in no time at all.

Most of all, we need to keep up our sunny sense of humor because no season has a corner on that sensation, not even summer!

Injured at Work?

When a worker suffers harm while on the job, they are supported by the worker's compensation insurance. Medical bills are taken care of and the worker is compensated for lost wages from missed days at work after their injuries.

Some employers are rigorous about employee wellness and others try to blame the employee for the accident. It is important that the employee not give up. Persistence is necessary; some insurance companies drag their heels to avoid paying out on their promises. others are happy to keep their reputation as trustworthy and reliable.

After being injured, the worker's priority is to restore their health and return to work as soon as possible. Many people with symptoms of pain and discomfort resulting from an injury or aggravated condition from a work injury may overuse are told to use prescription painkillers, especially opioids, through the worker's compensation system. As you've read in the news and in previous blog posts, the use of these drugs has increased tremendously over the past several years, regardless of their short-term benefit.

The United States consumes 80% of the world's pain medication while only having 6% of the world's population.

Even Non-Steroidal Anti-Inflammatory Drugs (NSAIDs) like Ibuprofen don't address the problem at its source and their use for relief as a long-term solution can be fatal. Fortunately, as the use of narcotic painkillers has risen, so too has the interest in more natural, alternative treatment options.

Vitamin D Tanning Beds: Separating the True from the False

All findings (below) are reported from this NEW STUDY that claims we should ignore the #1 cardinal rule in relation to sun exposure! A recent review of studies sought to review the health effects of solar radiation, tanning beds and vitamin D.

But since UV exposure has been suspected of causing skin cancer, many conventional health authorities still warn against it.

The researchers looked at data from different time periods for populations at different latitudes, with the aim at looking at the relative risk for cutaneous malignant melanoma associated with tanning bed use, vitamin D and UV effects.

They found that increased tanning bed use was NOT associated with melanoma.

According to the authors:

"Due to the fear of skin cancer, health authorities warn against sun and sunbed exposure. This policy, as well as the recommended vitamin d doses, may need revision."

and:

"... the overall health benefit of an improved vitamin d status may be more important than the possibly increased [cutaneous malignant melanoma] risk resulting from carefully increasing UV exposure."

In fact, Ivan Oransky, the editor of Reuters Health, has previously noted that the real risk of getting skin cancer from a tanning bed is less than three-tenths of one percent — and even then, this is likely only from those who habitually overexpose themselves.

Sun Exposure and Skin Cancer

The authors of the featured review state that while sun exposure is commonly assumed to be the main cause of cutaneous malignant melanoma (CMM) hereafter referred to simply as melanoma, the most lethal form of skin cancer — the matter is actually NOT "settled."

The theory is still under dispute, and in their analysis, they reviewed the arguments for and against causation.

Isn't Sun Exposure Linked with Cancer?

With a hint of irony, the authors state that "several factors are probably involved, as exemplified by a relationship sometimes found between gross domestic product and melanoma incidence." They also list a number of associations between sun exposure and melanoma found in the medical literature, such as:

- Intermittent sun exposure and severe sunburn in childhood are associated with an increased risk of melanoma

- Occupational exposure, such as farmers and fishermen, and regular weekend sun exposure are associated with decreased risk of melanoma

- Sun exposure appears to protect against melanoma on skin sites not exposed to sun light, and melanoma occurring on skin with large UV exposure has the best prognosis

- Patients with the highest blood levels of vitamin D have thinner melanoma and better survival prognosis than those with the lowest vitamin D levels.

Aren't Tanning Beds Dangerous?

So, what about tanning beds — are they more dangerous than regular sun exposure? As you may recall, the Senate's health-care overhaul bill now includes a 10 percent tax on tanning services to dissuade you from engaging in such "health-harming" activities; a move that is unquestionably short sighted and counterproductive considering the fact that vitamin D deficiency is rampant in the U.S.

Where tanning beds are concerned, the science is more conflicted, with some studies finding no detrimental impact from tanning beds on skin cancer rates while others have found that rates of skin cancer are higher in those using tanning beds than those who do not tan. The reason for these conflicting findings, the authors speculate, could very well be due to differences in UVA/UVB ratios and intensities between different types of tanning beds.

If Sun Exposure Increases Your Risk of Cancer, Just How Great is that Risk?

Even when looking at the research showing an increased risk for skin cancer from sun exposure, just how great is that risk? Ivan Oransky, M.D., editor of Reuters Health wrote an excellent commentary on this last year.

Each year, during the month of May, as the sun slowly begins to thaw away those winter blues, you start getting bombarded with Skin Cancer Awareness ads; all of which pitch the idea that the sun is your enemy. Many will include the statistic issued by the World Health Organization, which states that "use of sunbeds before the age of 35 is associated with a 75 percent increase in the risk of melanoma."

Sounds horrific, but how real is this threat?

"[W]hat does that really mean? Is it 75 percent greater than an already-high risk, or a tiny one?" Oransky writes.

"If you read the FDA's "*Indoor Tanning: The Risks of Ultraviolet Rays,*" or a number of other documents from the who and skin cancer foundations, you won't find your actual risk. That led AHCJ member Hiran Ratnayake to look into the issue in March for the (Wilmington, DE) news journal, after Delaware passed laws limiting teens' access to tanning salons. The 75 percent figure is based on a review of a number of studies, Ratnayake learned. the strongest such study was *one that followed more than 100,000 women over eight years.*

But as Ratnayake noted, that study "found that less than three-tenths of one percent who tanned frequently developed melanoma while less than two-tenths of one percent who didn't tan developed melanoma." That's actually about a 55 percent increase, but when the study was pooled with others, the average was a 75 percent increase.

In other words, even if the risk of melanoma was 75 percent greater than two-tenths of one percent, rather than 55 percent greater, it would still be far below one percent."

So, while statistically true, it's really misleading, and incites undue fear. By only presenting the relative risk increase (the 75 percent increase) they make the risk sound rather unreasonable. Meanwhile, your absolute risk of developing skin cancer from sun exposure is still, at worst, below one percent! And please remember, these highly distorted scare tactics fail to mention the benefits of the exposure, which radically reduce the dangers of the far more common, breast, prostate and colon cancers that are reduced.

Oransky explains the importance of understanding the difference between relative risk and absolute risk in his article:

"Absolute risk just tells you the chance of something happening, while relative risk tells you how that risk compares to another risk, as a ratio. If a risk doubles, for example, that's a relative risk of 2, or 200 percent. If it halves, it's 0.5, or 50 percent. Generally, when you're dealing with small absolute risks, as we are with melanoma, the relative risk differences will seem much greater than the absolute risk differences.

You can see how if someone is lobbying to ban something — or, in the case of a new drug, trying to show a dramatic effect — they would probably want to use the relative risk. ... so, when you read a study that says something doubles the risk of some terrible disease, ask: doubles from what to what?"

Tanning beds decrease ten times more cancers than they cause.

Another important factor to keep in mind is that vitamin D, ideally from sun exposure, may decrease your risk of many other cancers and chronic diseases.

According to the featured review:

"... it can be estimated that increased sun exposure to the Norwegian population might at worst result in 200-300 more melanoma deaths per year, but it would elevate the vitamin D status by about 25 nmol/l and might result in 4,000 fewer internal cancers and about 3,000 fewer cancer deaths overall.

The lack of sunlight exposure leads to more health problems than bone disease and increased risk of cancer. other benefits include protection against infectious diseases and non-cancerous diseases (diabetes, CVD, multiple sclerosis, and mental disorders)."

Overall, I believe the less than one percent risk of developing skin cancer from sun exposure or a tanning bed is well worth it, as increased vitamin D levels will protect you against so many other debilitating and lethal diseases and cancers... There's also compelling research showing that sun exposure will indeed protect you against melanoma — the most dangerous form of skin cancer.

Sun Exposure is the BEST Way to optimize Your Vitamin D Levels — it's intricately tied to healthy cholesterol and sulfur levels, making the recommendation to get your vitamin D from the sun all the more important.

In my view, a tanning bed comes in as a close second after natural sun exposure as the ideal way to optimize your vitamin D levels (as opposed to getting it from fortified food items or supplements).

In a recent interview, Dr. Stephanie Seneff explained how vitamin D — specifically from sun exposure — is intricately tied to healthy cholesterol and sulfur levels, making the recommendation to get your vitamin D from the sun all the more important.

Creating Space with Spinal Decompression Therapy

What Is Spinal Decompression Therapy?

Spinal decompression therapy is a modern, non-surgical traction procedure that effectively treats low back, neck, and radiating leg and arm pain. Spinal decompression therapy decompresses spinal discs and facet joints by utilizing traction, distraction, and body positioning.

Research to develop this procedure was conducted by prominent physicians, engineers and technicians at major teaching hospitals. Our SpineMED® decompression table is FDA approved and has been clinically proven to provide pain relief and decrease symptoms associated with herniated and/or bulging discs.

How Does it Work?

In nonsurgical spinal decompression therapy, the spine is stretched and relaxed intermittently in a controlled manner. The theory is that this process creates a negative *intradiscal* pressure (pressure within the disc itself), which is thought to have two potential benefits:

- Pulls the herniated or bulging disc material back into the disc.

- Promotes the passage of healing nutrients, into the disc and fosters a better healing environment.

During spinal decompression therapy for the low back (lumbar spine), patients remain clothed and lie on a motorized table, the lower half of which can move.

- A harness is placed around the hips and is attached to the lower table near the feet.

- The upper part of the table remains in a fixed position while the lower part, to which the patient is harnessed, slides back and forth to provide the traction and relaxation.

A set of pads is fastened around the hips and a fixed harness strap is tightened around the torso to prevent sliding down the table. Once positioned, a set amount of force (lbs.) is applied in a slow and controlled fashion to provide traction and relaxation over a series of cycles. The treatment protocol is a 30 minutes session.

The patient should not feel pain during or after the decompression therapy although they should feel stretch in the spine.

Who Qualifies?

This type of traction is very successful in relieving low back, neck pain, and radiating arm and leg pain. This space-giving therapy can be an effective treatment for:

- Herniated or Bulging
- Discs

- Sciatica

- Degenerative Disc

- Disease

- Post-surgical Patients

- Facet Syndrome

- Spinal Stenosis

What is the Research on Spinal Decompression Therapy?

Studies have shown that the spinal disc injury is responsible for a significant number of lumbar/leg pain and neck/arm pain syndromes. Excessive compression forces from daily activities increases internal spinal disc pressure which can lead to spinal disc protrusion, herniation, and bulging of disc material.

While spinal decompression therapy may be recommended as a potential treatment for a variety of lower back pain conditions, as with all lower back pain treatments, it is the patient's decision whether or not to have the treatment.

Recent research has shown that 86% of the 219 patients who completed decompression therapy reported immediate resolution of symptoms, while 84% remained pain-free 90 days post-treatment. Physical examination findings showed improvement in 92% of the 219 patients and remained intact in 89% of these patients 90 days after treatment (Gionis, Thomas MD; Groteke, Eric DC. *Surgical Alternatives: Spinal Decompression. Orthopedic Technology Review. 2003; 6 (5)*, 1-9.

No "Cocooning": Are We Ever Too Old to Benefit from Chiropractic Care?

I say, "Not even close!" Here is the research we have uncovered as to why.

Did you know that in the US alone nearly 20% of the population will be 65 or older by 2030? Chiropractic is one of the most frequently utilized types of complementary and alternative care by older adults, used by an estimated 5% of older adults in the U.S. annually.

According to author Paul E. Dougherty, author of *The Role of Chiropractic Care in Older Adults*:

An estimated 14% of patients treated by doctors of chiropractic (DCs) are 65 and older. The most common reason for an older adult to see a DC is musculoskeletal pain, most often lower back pain. Although the most common reason for older adults seeking chiropractic care is for musculoskeletal symptoms, DCs may also provide a diverse range of services to these patients.

Regardless of your age, chiropractic care can help improve mobility and maintain vitality. With growing concerns about over-medication and the side effects of combining various prescription drugs, safe, natural chiropractic care is growing in popularity.

As we age, we atrophy unless we adjust ourselves to new ways of living. As an example of this, slouching can significantly hinder the joints. Therefore, aging adults must make it a priority to stand and sit up straight in order to protect their joints in the knees and neck. Good posture is also essential when elders are lifting and carrying objects because a lopsided posture adds stress to the joints.

Restoring better spinal function can also bring flexibility, endurance, and appetite. With even the smallest adjustments, people report improvement with arthritic symptoms, posture, muscular pain, and other chronic ailments often associated with the aging process such as elimination and sexual function.

I have been able to amass several findings that may inspire older adults to consider other benefits of chiropractic care. The quote chiropractic researcher Dr. Vic Naumov:

- 44% of those who used chiropractic care reported having arthritis compared with 66% in the non-chiropractic care group

- those who used chiropractic care were more likely to do strenuous levels of exercise

- at three years follow-up, less than 5% of those who used chiropractic care lived in a nursing home while a staggering 48% of those who did not use chiropractic care did live in a nursing home

- at three years follow-up, only 26% of those who used chiropractic care were hospitalized compared with 48% of those in the non-chiropractic group

The adjusting technique used by your chiropractor will be modified for maximum comfort and results. There is no need for seniors to suffer needlessly. Chiropractic provides amazing benefits and has an outstanding record of safety and effectiveness.

Heads Up: Can Chiropractic Care Treat Concussions?

What is a Concussion?

Injuries to the head and neck during sports, accidents, and other traumatic events are common. Two of the most frequently occurring conditions in the head and neck area are whiplash (a particular neck injury from high velocity forces) and concussion (a closed-head injury, sometimes called mild traumatic brain injury). These two injuries could both occur during the same incident, but not always in ways that are immediately obvious. Because I explore whiplash more thoroughly in another essay on this website, I'm choosing here to focus on concussion.

A concussion is a type of traumatic brain injury (TBI) caused by a bump, blow, or jolt to the head or by a hit to the body that causes the head and brain to move rapidly back and forth.

According to the Centers for Disease Control and Prevention (CDCP), between 2001 and 2009, an estimated 173,285 people under age 19 were treated in hospital emergency rooms for concussions related to sports and recreation activities. Other causes include car and bicycle accidents, work-related injuries, falls, and fights.

A hard blow to the head can shake the brain inside the skull, resulting in bruising, broken blood vessels, or nerve damage to the brain. There no outward bleeding or opening in the skull, it could result in a closed brain injury. An open brain injury is when an object penetrates the skull and goes into the brain.

How Can You Tell If You Have Had a Concussion?

Concussions are usually not life threatening. Even so, their effects can be serious. Concussive symptoms usually fall in one of four categories:

- Thinking/remembering
- Physical

- Emotional/mood

- Sleep

Red Flags

- Any difficulty walking

- Any loss of consciousness, confusion, or significant agitation

- One pupil (the black part in the middle of the eye) larger than the other

- Loss of ability to identify people, places, the date, or self

- Loss of motion or sensation, weakness, numbness or loss of coordination

- Persistent, worsening headache

- Repeated vomiting

- Slurred speech or difficulty with expression

- Seizures

- Kids will not stop crying and cannot be consoled

- Kids will not nurse or eat

Get to the ER right away if you have any of these danger signs after any type of head injury, no matter how minor it may seem.

What Do Chiropractors Do for People with Concussions?

Most medical journals will say, "There are no treatments for concussions other than prevention of an additional injury. "

Any blow to the head will cause a misalignment of the cervical spine (a symptom similar to whiplash). A chiropractor can evaluate whether you demonstrate signs of neck injuries commonly associated with concussions and provide you with relief of neck pain and headaches.

According to the literature reviews, one of the most important recommendations that a chiropractor will tell you what to do for concussion is this: If you or your loved one is in sports and suffers a blow to the head, and/or experiences signs of a concussion, do not let them continue playing the sport. He or she needs to rest until totally healed from the concussion. Only after symptoms subside is it time to get back into the game. Ease into the sports play again. Don't expect to jump back in, full force. This will prevent the return of symptoms.

Additional guidelines your chiropractor will give you for concussion include no alcohol, recreational drugs, aspirin, anti-inflammatory medications, and sleep agents should be consumed. Use Tylenol for pain, if necessary. By all means, do not drive until you can return to the sport.

Chiropractors can help with a range of other sports injuries, and one study even found that it was the most effective conservative method for reducing sports-related back pain.

Straighten Up: Posture and Overall Health

What Is Posture All About?

Posture is not something you "do" it is something you "have" as a result of the bones in your body (mostly in your spine) being stacked correctly. If this is the case, your body just stays upright without muscular effort. Bad posture therefore has nothing to do with laziness, with weak muscles, or with tight ligaments.

The best way to check if any traditional bodywork method has made a real structural correction is to "breathe in, breathe out, let your body relax and slump". If you are still slumping after treatment by a chiropractor, osteopath, physical therapist, or other bodywork professional, structural correction did not actually occur. Immediately after the first visit, your shoulders should stay upright and back, and you should notice a difference to your breathing. If that is not the case, structural correction did not occur; things got moved around, but not actually corrected.

Posture is not something you "do" it is something you "have" as a result of the bones in your body being stacked correctly.

What Can Our Posture Tell Us?

Posture is a window to our overall health. Over time, poor posture may be caused by habits from everyday activities such as sitting in office chairs, staring at the computer, staring at our smartphones, carrying a backpack or purse over the same shoulder year after year, driving, prolonged standing, attending to small children, or even sleeping.

Correct posture is a simple but very important way to keep the many intricate structures in the back and spine healthy. It is much more than cosmetic — good posture and back support are critical to reducing the incidence and levels of back pain and neck pain.

Without good posture, our nervous system will not function optimally because structure dictates function. Three curves must be present in our spine in order to have good health. When one of these curves is lost or reversed, we will distribute our weight incorrectly and cause pain syndromes.

How Do We Assess Our Posture?

When I give a Living Well workshop, I have the attendants pair up with their classmates for a "photo opp." I recommend they remove their outer layers of clothing for the most visible measurement. I ask each attendant to take three full-body photos of each other with their smartphones — one from the front, one from the back and one from the side. I say, "relax your muscles and stand as tall as you can, feet hip-width apart." I then invite them to diagnose the following posture problems, saying:

- Look at your partner's ear. If it's in front of the midpoint of their shoulder, their head is too far forward.

- Can you see their shoulder blade? That means their back is too rounded.

- If their hips tilt forward and they have a belly pooch (even if they don't have an ounce of fat on their body) and their lower spine is arched significantly, this means they have an anterior pelvic tilt.

- Look at your neighbor's shoulders. One shouldn't appear higher than the other.

- Check out their kneecaps. Do they point inward, causing their knees to touch when their legs are straightened?

- See if they're duck-footed. Their toes will point outward more than 10 degrees.

What Causes It?

The most common cause of poor posture is lack of regular exercise. The second most common cause is going long periods of time spent hunched over at a desk or a smartphone. As a result, muscles and wrappings of muscle and connective tissue in the body, called fascia, shorten. As well as make us look hunched over, and much older than our years. These habits can limit our ability to move, reducing the effectiveness of the diaphragm which reduces oxygenation, and impairs the digestive system. This leads to problems such as fatigue, headaches, poor concentration and, of course, immobility, inflexibility and stiffness.

What Can Be Done to Correct It?

At Living Well Chiropractic:

- We treat and repair the underlying cause of your symptoms.

- We correct your body structure so well that your posture is automatically corrected and realigned.

- As your body's structure is corrected your body will untwist from previous injuries which are still there but compensated for (like wear and tear).

We always document progress with before and after pictures which let you see the changes for yourself and offer an objectively measurable way to quantify results. As your structure gets corrected, you will find yourself once again engaging in activities that you hadn't been able to carry out for years or decades.

We turn the clock back on bodies and reverse all kinds of structural and postural problems which conventional wisdom attributes to "normal, age-related wear and tear." Our work together can be lasting when we practice consistent wellness habits. This progress is measurable over time.

What Can Be Done to Prevent It?

Improving our posture can be done with the help of good chiropractic care. We can make progress when we learn new methods to sit at our desks, use any equipment we use in an ergonomic way (i.e., when lifting or using a keyboard and mouse) and by the way we hold ourselves when standing.

Uptight: Can Stress Be Lessened with Chiropractic Care?

What is Stress?

Stress is a specific response by the body to a stimulus, i.e., fear or pain, that disturbs or interferes with the normal physiological equilibrium of an organism. We at Living Well Chiropractic perceive stress from four basic sources: our environment, our body, our emotions and by exposure to various chemicals.

I like to refer to them as "The Three T's — Thoughts, Traumas and Toxins." We'll go deeper into each in a moment, but regardless of the source of the stress, the physiological response by the body is the same. Stress can manifest differently for everyone, with the most common symptoms being; headaches, fatigue, sleep problems, pain, digestive issues and/or irritability/mood swings.

Stress is a reality of modern living. Especially in Western Society, where more and more of us are working longer hours and the media is constantly overloading our senses with the latest tragedy, it's easy to see why many people experience anxiety levels ranging from mild to acute.

According to the latest statistics, stress is the leading cause of 80% of all human illness and disease. Three out of four doctor's visits each day are for stress-related ailments. Stress increases heart disease 40%, heart attack 25%, and stroke 50%. Forty-percent of stressed people overeat or eat unhealthy foods. Forty-four percent of stressed people lose sleep every night.

Stress-related ailments cost the nation $300 billion dollars every year in medical bills and lost productivity.

Where is a majority of the stress stored?

Stress is often stored in one of the largest muscles in our body, the psoas (pronounced Sew-Az). This muscle stretches from our lower trunk through our hips into the top of our thighs, it is used for core stability and the fight flight reflex. Even witnessing a violent scene in a movie will ignite our brain to send signals our body to respond by releasing epinephrine (adrenaline).

The muscle that is most central to our fight/flight response is the psoas. When we don't respond, these stress hormones go unspent and become stored in the body. This can bring many health problems including insomnia, lowered immune system, anxiety, eating disorders, depression, and living in a constant state of fear or alert.

The good news is that chiropractic care can help us manage our stress levels and treat it at its source. Read on to see how...

How We React to Stress

As we discussed above, stress comes in three main forms. Our Thoughts — relationship problems, financial issues, loss of a loved one. Traumas — these can be macro-traumas like a car accident or slip and fall, or they can be micro-traumas like repetitively doing the same thing (i.e. working at a computer for long hours, bending and lifting throughout the day, etc.). Finally, there are Toxins — these are things we are exposed to either in the air or internally. For example, the things we eat. If we ingest too much of the bad foods (sugars, processed foods, fried foods) and not enough of the good foods (fruits, vegetables, protein), this can create stress to the gut by causing inflammation and possible damage to the lining of the intestines due to malnutrition. So, whether the stressor is due to poor nutrition, poor sleep and/or physical injury, our bodies release different hormones such as cortisol and adrenaline when we're stressed to help us have quick energy to cope.

PHYSICAL STRESS can be born of, or even lead to, poor nutrition, poor sleep, and physical injury. Our bodies release adrenaline when we're stressed to help us have quick energy to cope. Whether the stress is physical danger, like being chased by a gorilla, or emotional, such as a break-up, death of a loved one or job loss, the physical effects of adrenaline in the body (especially for long periods) is wearing. Given all this, it's easy to see how stress causes excessive wear and damage that leaves us exhausted. Such burn out leads us to reaching for foods and substances to relax or give us a boost to keep going. By adding these chemicals, we've just doubled the amount of manageable stress.

For example: when we're in a panic we become saturated with stress hormones like adrenaline, cortisol, norepinephrine, this saturation results in a "shut down" response; a pattern that creates not only sleep deprivation and exhaustion but a sluggish metabolism. Experts agree, when you're not balanced, you are more likely to shovel in quick energy, chemically-manufactured, high-sugar foods and skip workouts. When amped up or exhausted (same hormonal coin), who wants to eat whole foods, move more intentionally, or even workout?

How Does Stress Affect Our Nervous System?

A threat is perceived

The autonomic nervous system automatically puts body on alert.

The adrenal cortex automatically releases stress hormones.

The heart automatically beats harder and more rapidly.

Breathing automatically becomes more rapid.

Thyroid gland automatically stimulates the metabolism.

Larger muscles automatically receive more oxygenated blood.

The important thing to take away is that the fight or flight response is an automatic response. It is a much-needed response mechanism to acute stressors. The autonomic nervous system is responsible for organ, gland and hormonal function has two parts. They serve like an on/off switch. The sympathetic part is the fight or flight portion, and the parasympathetic part is the rest and digest portion. However, if our nervous system is unable to suppress the fight or flight response, we will remain in a heightened, over-stimulated state. The longer we are in this "sympathetic" state, the more likely we are to suffer with fatigue and burnout of the adrenal glands which are the primary stress glands in our body.

EMOTIONAL STRESS is more difficult to define. It encompasses our reactions, in thought and emotion, to environmental and physical stressors. Receiving criticism, for example, is devastating to some, while others seem unaffected.

How do you know if what you're feeling is too much? Maybe you're just having a bad day or perhaps a rough few weeks. Are you just feeling down, a little anxious, irritable or are you feeling one breath away from the "last straw"?

If so, you may be surprised to learn it's quite common; doctors say it's part of the human condition. Charles Goodstein, MD, clinical professor of psychiatry at NYU Medical Center in New York City says, "The presence of anxiety, of a depressive mood or of a conflict within the mind, does not stamp any individual as having a psychological problem because, as a matter of fact, these qualities are indigenous to the species." But if living on the "last straw" has more or less become your way of life, experts say there's something on your mind that is crying out for your attention. The key is how often you are feeling this sense of distress, how bad it gets, and how long it lasts; that is what can help determine the seriousness of your situation.

ENVIRONMENTAL STRESS includes noise, weather, physical threats, time pressures and performance standards. Holidays or special milestone events can leave both host and guest feeling exhausted by merely anticipating what goes into the "big day" (or season)! Expectations can be all out of proportion setting up even greater disappointments. But even with greater awareness of these pitfalls, year after year, our "fight or flight" response to stress kicks in.

Everyday life is also full of environmental stressors that cause minor irritations. If you use an alarm clock to wake up, the loud noise from your alarm is an environmental stressor. Extreme temperatures are also environmental stressors and can lead to discomfort. Other common environmental stressors include:

- Noise
- Crowding
- Air quality
- Overstimulating light/prolonged exposure to dark
- Natural disasters
- Social tensions among groups (whether in our midst or in the world at large)
- War and other human-made disasters

Recent research has linked extreme temperatures, crowding, and noise with increased levels of discomfort and aggression. Studies have also shown that crime rates are higher during those hot summer days. Exposure to light can improve your mood and decrease fatigue, while prolonged exposure to darkness can interfere with sleep patterns and lead to symptoms of depression.

The World Health Organization (WHO) has acknowledged environmental pollution as the underlying cause in nearly 80% of all chronic degenerative diseases. Toxic chemicals and metals have the potential to negatively impact every biological function occurring within your body.

CHEMICAL STRESS: Doctors from the University of California and the Boston Medical Center have released findings, linking common chemical pollutants to at least 200 different human diseases. Data from hundreds of research studies over the years has shown strong correlations between various common chemical stresses and a wide range of diseases.

These include, but are not limited to:

- asthma
- testicular atrophy
- cerebral palsy
- kidney disease
- heart disease
- hypertension
- diabetes

There are thousands of chemicals, how could we possibly discuss them all?

We cannot, nor could we pronounce them all, but here is a sample of the various types of chemicals that pollute our earth and our bodies.

- Industrial chemicals
- Chlorinated solvents
- Artificial, processed or genetically-modified (GMO) foods

- Pesticides

- Dyes

- Pharmaceuticals

- Synthetic Hormones

- And MORE...

What Does Chiropractic Care Offer to Transform Stress Patterns?

While chiropractic care does not transform your outside stressors, studies show that chiropractic care may be effective at relieving stress. Much of the work that a chiropractor does is with the spine, the root of the nervous system. Your body is constantly adapting to both its external environment as well as its internal environment. We call this G.A.P. or General Adaptation Potential. The greater your GAP, the greater the body's ability to handle stress. The nervous system is directly responsible for managing stressors. If there is spinal subluxation, the nervous system's ability to function optimally is blocked and you become less equipped to handle stress. Each chiropractic adjustment reduces interference to the nervous system and improves function. As our function increases, so does the capability to cope with external stressors. Because stress often triggers symptoms in the nervous system, spinal manipulation or adjustments can help restore balance to the nervous system and hormonal system.

Chiropractic focuses on the spine, which is the root of the nervous system. One of the effects of chronic stress is muscle tension and contraction, which can lead to uneven pressure on the skeleton, which in turn leads to subluxations. By determining which part of the nervous system is functioning improperly, the chiropractic adjustment can be performed to influence the sympathetic or parasympathetic branch.

Adjustments reduce the subluxations which help ease muscle tension and decrease the stress to the skeleton. Reducing subluxations balances the spine and improves the function of the nervous system by eliminating interference. Our nerves, work much like a garden hose that is crimped and only allows a trickle of water to flow. When you remove the crimp, you have increased flow of water.

Research suggests that up to 80 percent of all illness is related to stress, which starts with minor symptoms such as backache, headache, and fatigue. To put it simply, chiropractic adjustments to the spine, as well as other muscles and joints, may actually help tell the nervous system to relax and cause the stress response to fade.

At Living Well Chiropractic, we believe we have multiple methods to share that foster a return to balance no matter what is happening within or outside of us. Relaxation techniques, meditation and contemplation, hypnosis and similar approaches can all have a strong mediating effect on stress.

Here are three helpful stress management tips from Living Well:

1. Know that stress will come — so, know your "hot buttons" or "triggers" and know who pushes them.

2. Take 10 minutes each night to organize things for the next day and be reasonable in what you can achieve in one day.

3. Finally, proceed through the day in confidence and stay focused.

After decades of research, it is clear that the negative effects associated with stress are real. Although you may not always be able to avoid stressful situations, there are a number of things that you can do to reduce the effect that stress has on your body. The first is relaxation.

Just as each individual with show signs of stress differently, each individual needs to figure out their own path to relaxation. Below are four of the most common ways to relieve stress naturally:

Relaxed Breathing

Practice this basic four-by-four or box technique twice a day, every day, and whenever you feel tense. Follow these steps:

- Inhale. With your mouth closed and your shoulders relaxed, inhale as slowly and deeply as you can to the count of four. As you do that, push your stomach out. Allow the air to fill your diaphragm.

- Hold. Keep the air in your lungs as you slowly count to four.

- Exhale. Release the air through your mouth as you slowly count to four.

- Hold. Keep the air in your lungs as you slowly count to four.

- Repeat the inhale-hold-exhale-hold cycle four times.

Progressive Muscle Relaxation

The goal of progressive muscle relaxation is to reduce the tension in your muscles. First, find a quiet place where you'll be free from interruption. Loosen tight clothing and remove your glasses or contacts if you'd like.

Tense each muscle group for at least five seconds and then relax for at least 30 seconds. Repeat before moving to the next muscle group.

- Upper part of your face. Lift your eyebrows toward the ceiling, feeling the tension in your forehead and scalp. Relax. Repeat.

- Central part of your face. Squint your eyes tightly and wrinkle your nose and mouth, feeling the tension in the center of your face. Relax. Repeat.

- Lower part of your face. Clench your teeth and pull back the corners of your mouth toward your ears. Show your teeth like a snarling dog. Relax. Repeat.

- Neck. Gently touch your chin to your chest. Feel the pull in the back of your neck as it spreads into your head. Relax. Repeat.

- Shoulders. Pull your shoulders up toward your ears, feeling the tension in your shoulders, head, neck and upper back. Relax. Repeat.

- Upper arms. Pull your arms back and press your elbows in toward the sides of your body. Try not to tense your lower arms. Feel the tension in your arms, shoulders and into your back. Relax. Repeat.

- Hands and lower arms. Make a tight fist and pull up your wrists. Feel the tension in your hands, knuckles and lower arms. Relax. Repeat.

- Chest, shoulders and upper back. Pull your shoulders back as if you're trying to make your shoulder blades touch. Relax. Repeat.

- Stomach. Pull your stomach in toward your spine, tightening your abdominal muscles. Relax. Repeat.

- Upper legs. Squeeze your knees together and lift your legs up off the chair or from wherever you're relaxing. Feel the tension in your thighs. Relax. Repeat.

- Lower legs. Raise your feet toward the ceiling while flexing them toward your body. Feel the tension in your calves. Relax. Repeat.

- Feet. Turn your feet inward and curl your toes up and out. Relax. Repeat.

Perform progressive muscle relaxation at least once or twice each day to get the maximum benefit. Each session should last about 10 minutes.

Listen to Soothing Sounds

If you have about 10 minutes and a quiet room, you can take a mental vacation almost anytime. We in the Pacific Northwest are blessed to have multiple locations to get quiet. Even if we can't escape to the landscapes of mountains, rivers, lakes, parks or the Pacific Ocean, we can listen to these sounds by downloading "the sounds of nature" apps on our smart phones

- Soothing nature sounds help us concentrate in a one-pointed way, leaving our worries behind.

- Guided meditation apps educate us on stress reduction or take us to a peaceful place.

- Music has the power to affect our thoughts and feelings. Soft, soothing music can help us relax and lower our stress levels.

No one app works for everyone, so try several to find which works best for you. When possible, listen to samples or ask your friends or a trusted professional for recommendations.

Exercise

Exercise is a good way to relieve pent-up energy and tension. It also helps us get in better shape, which makes us feel better overall. By getting physically active, we decrease our levels of anxiety and stress and elevate our moods. Numerous studies have shown that people who begin exercise programs, either at home or at work, demonstrate a marked improvement in their ability to concentrate, are able to sleep better, suffer from fewer illnesses, suffer from less pain and report a much higher quality of life than those who do not exercise. This is even true of people who had not begun an exercise program until they were in their 40s, 50s, 60s or even 70s. So, if you want to feel better and improve your quality of life, get active!

These techniques provide tools that allow us gain greater control over reactions to stress, and therefore reduce the overall effects of all three forms of stress (environmental, physical or emotional).

More than Aches and Pains: How Does Chiropractic Care Treat Fibromyalgia?

What is Fibromyalgia?

Fibromyalgia (FM) causes chronic pain throughout the body as well as sensitivity to pressure. Sufferers of this syndrome often also experience intense fatigue, trouble sleeping and stiff joints. Due to these symptoms, those with fibromyalgia usually also experience anxiety and depression. Since there is no real cure for this disorder in the traditional medical world, it is necessary to control the symptoms to allow those with fibromyalgia to live a normal, pain-free life.

According to the National Fibromyalgia Association the painful disorder affects approximately 10 million individuals, mostly women, in the United States alone. Researchers believe that fibromyalgia amplifies pain sensations by altering the way the brain processes pain signals.

Most people suffer pain in ways that only their closest loved ones see. Many are blamed as being hypochondriacs, suffering from Munchausen Syndrome or "just" depressed. The average health professional may know a little bit about "fibromyalgia pain" – as if it were a singular sensation – but for sufferers, several kinds of pain exist throughout their bodies.

What Causes Fibromyalgia?

Medical science is yet to discover the cause for this condition. Because there are so many different symptoms associated with fibromyalgia, there are just as many theories for what causes it. Since those with FM often experience an altered mood – such as depression – many experts focus on the psychological aspect of the disease. Others feel that FM is more a physiological entity and has its origins in physical trauma or chronic postural alterations. Some suggest that FM is a central nervous system disorder, with imbalances in neurochemicals — since those with FM are hypersensitive to even the slightest stimuli. They often have a pain response to normally non-painful pressure or activity. It's not out of the question that a combination of psychological and physical triggers can result in the onset of many of FM symptoms. Still, many medical professionals refer patients to psychotherapists or pain-managing pharmaceuticals.

What do our patients say?

When they first sought treatment, they learned that fibromyalgia pain has been medically defined as followed:

Hyperalgesia: 'Hyper' *huper* from Ancient Greek (over), *-algesia* from Greek (pain) is an increased sensitivity to pain, which may be caused by damage to nociceptors or peripheral nerves. Temporary increased sensitivity to pain which may also emerge as an evolved response to infection.

Allodynia: Ancient Greek *állos* (other) and *odúne* "pain") refers to central pain sensitization (increased response of neurons) following painful, often repetitive, stimulation. Allodynia can lead to the triggering of a pain response from stimuli which do not normally provoke pain. Temperature or physical stimuli can provoke allodynia, which may feel like a burning sensation, and it often occurs after injury to a site. Allodynia is different from Hyperalgesia, an extreme, exaggerated reaction to a stimulus which is normally painful.

Painful Paresthesia: a sensation of tingling, tickling, pricking, or burning of a person's skin with no apparent physical cause. The manifestation of a paresthesia may be transient or chronic. The most familiar kind of paresthesia is the sensation known as "pins and needles" or of a limb "falling asleep."

Types of Pain Experientially Defined

My Living Well patients describe their FM sensations in the following terms:

- Feeling stabbed with pins and needles (like a voodoo doll)

- Matches being out on skin

- Walking through peanut butter

- Easily Rattled Nerves

Certain things tend to put the body on edge, jumpy, and feeling rattled. I'm told it emerges all over, and sometimes causes nauseous, dizzy and anxious. Things that rattle generally involve sensory or emotional overload, such as:

- Certain sounds (repetitive, loud, shrill, grating);

- Visual chaos (crowds, flashing lights, busy patterns);

- Stressful situations (busy traffic, confrontations, fibro-fog induced confusion or disorientation).

Living with Pain vs. Transforming the Pain

I've seen promising results in our patients suffering from fibromyalgia. We've seen them experience less back, neck and leg pain. Many fibromyalgia sufferers have what is called upper cervical spinal stenosis. This is when the upper spine coverings become compressed, causing severe pain. At Living Well, we have a SpineMED® decompression table that patients say the compression is released. When the spine is better aligned, pain levels go down.

There have been many studies done that analyze whether chiropractic treatment is providing real help to those suffering from fibromyalgia. One in particular was conducted in 1985, when 81 fibromyalgia patients were asked what type of treatment they thought best helped relieve their pain levels. Many opted for chiropractic, claiming it was the best at managing their body aches. Not only does chiropractic help lower pain, but it also is able to allow sufferers to sleep better and experience less fatigued during the day.

We believe that chiropractic care offers an especially good option for those looking for a way to get all-natural relief without the use of medications.

Fibromyalgia is a widely misunderstood and often misdiagnosed chronic disorder. Living with the symptoms is unnecessary. For more information, please feel free to ask via LivingWellBainbridge.com. It could put you on the path to living a pain-free life. If the condition is not diagnosed and treated early, symptoms can go on indefinitely, or they may disappear for months and then recur.

Besides Chiropractic Care What Else Can Be Done for Patients?

Besides mild or mildly-aggressive "hands on" chiropractic manipulation, many chiropractors use other methods to foster healing from and correction for spinal misalignment.

The Activator: The Activator Method Chiropractic Technique (AMCT) is a chiropractic treatment method and device created by Arlan Fuhr as an alternative to manual manipulation of the spine or extremity joints. The device is categorized as a mechanical force manual assisted (MFMA) instrument which is generally regarded as a softer chiropractic treatment technique.

Impulse: This technique uses tools that deliver gentle chiropractic adjustments to the spinal joints and extremities to relieve them of pain. Controlled thrusts are applied precisely on the desired area and it restores function as well. It does not cause any popping sound. It is effective and extremely safe for patients of all ages.

Rapid Release Treatment: This technique uses unique hand-held instrument which offers a specialized form of massage. It helps the chiropractor identify areas of restriction and break up the scar tissue. The instrument scans and detects the injured tissue where cross-fiction massage rubs against it. It increases the blood flow in the area and promotes the healing process. In some cases, mild inflammation can occur.

Pro-Adjuster: It uses sophisticated computerized analysis for detecting the problem areas and the pro-adjuster tool uses resonant force impulses on the affected areas. It helps in relieving pressure on the nervous system and promotes faster healing. It restores nerve's ability to transmit signals to and from the brain.

Osteo-Vibe: This "whole body vibration" (WBV) technique use machines that pair gravity and resistance with the transmission of low frequency vibrations to the human body, resulting in several positive effects including increases in: muscle power and strength, tone, circulation, bone density, balance and flexibility. Users also report lack of injury because of the machines ability to "warm up" the body, as well as an after-sport recovery aid. My daughters Kailey and Kori give an example of how these machines work.

Pierce-Stillwagon: This technique uses a drop table and a prone or sitting instrument that helps in supine or prone pelvic adjustments. Additionally, X-ray analysis can be used for making better clinical decisions regarding the spinal levels to adjust.

Decompression Table: Spinal decompression, also known as mechanical traction, has different forms. One way is to harness patients to a table on their stomachs or backs and apply static or intermittent pull to stretch the spine. Depending on the patient's condition, the health care professional adjusts the amount of time, the degree of pull and the angle of the traction. It can also be applied with heat or ice.

The best chiropractors teach (and learn from) patients other techniques to promote healing...

Light Exercise: According to the National Academy of Sports Medicine "Light Exercise" includes activities that do not cause you to break a sweat or produce shortness of breath. An example would be a leisurely walk or casual bike ride. Moderate exercise is exercise which causes you to break out in a light to moderate sweat or makes it difficult to carry on a long conversation. Good examples would be a brisk walk, hiking on a nature trail, performing chores around the house.

Therapeutic Massage: This form of massage incorporates a variety of advanced modalities that enhance the body's natural restorative functioning. Light to firm touch is used to release tension, relax muscles, increase blood and lymph circulation, and can impart a sense of calm.

Nutrition Advice: Good nutrition consultants can help you come up with a lifestyle plan that works for you. We at Living Well believe your lifestyle adjustments should be specific, measurable and do-able AND, most important, you should have a part in planning it. They should also guide you through the steps and help you realize things about your own eating habits that you may need to alter, i.e., how pre-prepared meal plans may come into play. Some chiropractors recommend nutritional supplements — vitamins and minerals.

New patients at Living Well undergo a first visit orthopedic and neurological examination. After completion of the evaluation, the patient is able to receive the first adjustment that same day provided no contraindications to care are found during the exam. For those who are not aware, an adjustment is the process by which a chiropractor introduces motion into spinal and other joints in the body to help restore their proper mobility and alignment.

When Do Chiropractors Recommend Outside Help?

There are more conditions than imagined respond to chiropractic help. But sometimes, patients don't improve with treatment. Good chiropractors do everything in their power to help their patients feel better as fast as possible with as few chiropractic treatments as necessary, ultimately reducing care to an as-needed follow-up plan. They also give advice on how to avoid future problems by evaluating lifestyle activities, ergonomics, posture, orthotics. Proactive recommendations include exercises and stretches; ergonomic tools like back supports, belts, or pillows; home rehabilitation tools like foam roller, elastic bands; orthotics; and/or dietary supplements.

In general, in the absence of progressive worsening of a condition during chiropractic care, a common chiropractic program is three times per week for 2 to 4 weeks, followed by a re-evaluation.

After the re-evaluation, an ethical chiropractor will refer the patient to another kind of help that may be a better fit for them.

Can Arthritis Be Treated with Chiropractic Care?

What is Arthritis?

Arthritis literally means "joint inflammation" but it is used as a collective term for a complex family of musculoskeletal (muscle and skeleton) disorders that include over 100 different diseases or conditions.

The Arthritis Foundation, a non-profit organization in the US, estimates that there are 53 million Americans living with arthritis.

Although the image that comes to mind when discussing arthritis is an older adult, arthritis can affect people of any age. In fact, two-thirds of the cases of arthritis are found in adults under the age of 65, and 300,000 children in the U.S. have arthritis. Symptoms of rheumatoid arthritis and osteoarthritis often overlap but have some fundamental differences and require different treatments.

Many people confide in me, "The orthopedist told me the disc in my neck or low back is worn down because of my age." His response is: "Well, how old are the other discs in your spine?"

What's the Difference Between the Two Major Types?

Rheumatoid Arthritis (RA)

Joint inflammation from Rheumatoid Arthritis (RA) is different from Osteoarthritis though both come with pain, warmth, and swelling. In Rheumatoid Arthritis, the inflammation is typically symmetrical, occurring on both sides of the body at the same time (such as the wrists, knees, or hands). Other symptoms of RA include joint stiffness, particularly in the morning or after periods of inactivity; ongoing fatigue, and low-grade fever. Symptoms typically develop gradually over years, but they can come on rapidly for some people.

A healthy immune system is protective. It generates internal inflammation to get rid of infection and prevent disease. But the immune system can go awry, mistakenly attacking the joints with uncontrolled inflammation, potentially causing joint erosion and may damage internal organs, eyes and other parts of the body. Researchers believe that a combination of genetics and environmental factors can trigger this autoimmunity. Smoking is an example of an environmental risk factor that can trigger rheumatoid arthritis in people with certain genes.

With autoimmune and inflammatory types of arthritis, early diagnosis and aggressive treatment is critical. Slowing disease activity can help minimize or even prevent permanent joint damage. Remission is the goal and in the dominant practice in medicine is often to prescribe the use of one or more medications known as disease-modifying anti-rheumatic drugs (DMARDs). The goal of treatment of both RA and Osteoarthritis is to reduce pain, improve function, and prevent further joint damage. If the symptoms of arthritis are not arrested, the source of the pain may have been misidentified.

Osteoarthritis (OA)

In most cases, osteoarthritis develops in the weight-bearing joints of the knees, hips, or spine. It's also common in the fingers. Other joints such as the elbow, wrist, and ankle are usually not affected, unless an injury is involved.

Also called "wear and tear" arthritis or degenerative joint disease, osteoarthritis (OA) is the progressive breakdown of the joints' natural shock absorbers. This can cause discomfort when you use the affected joints — perhaps an ache when you bend at the hips or knees, or sore fingers when you type. Most people over 60 have some degree of OA, but it also affects people in their 20s and 30s.

The estimated 27 million people in the U.S. who have osteoarthritis include all ethnic and socioeconomic backgrounds. But some people are more likely to develop OA than others. Athletes and people with jobs that require a lot of repetitive motion are at higher risk because of injuries and stress on joints. Obesity and aging also increase risk.

Osteoarthritis tends to strike weight bearing joints in the knees and hips or spine. But it can develop in any joint where cartilage wears away and the bones lose their cushioning. The symptoms of osteoarthritis tend to develop slowly. Many notice pain or soreness when they've been inactive for a prolonged period. The affected joints may also be stiff or creaky.

Typically, osteoarthritis leads to morning stiffness that resolves in 30 minutes. When it affects the hands, some people develop bony enlargements in the fingers, which may or may not cause pain. Other joints such as the elbow, wrist, and ankle are usually not affected, unless an injury is involved.

Unlike rheumatoid arthritis, osteoarthritis does not affect the body's organs or cause illness. But it can lead to deformities that take a toll on mobility. Severe loss of cartilage in the knee joints can cause the knees to curve out, creating a bow-legged appearance (shown on the left). Bony spurs along the spine (shown on the right) can irritate nerves, leading to pain, numbness, or tingling in some parts of the body.

What Can Be Done About Arthritis?

There are many things that can be done to preserve joint function, mobility and quality of life. Learning about the disease and treatment options, making time for physical activity and maintaining a healthy weight are essential. Therapeutic massage is also known to give relief, sometimes in long lasting ways. But, arthritis is a commonly misunderstood disease and it is vital to have the source of the pain identified.

Can Diet Help?

From a natural, holistic perspective, the foods we eat play a significant role in inflammatory responses. David Getoff, vice president of the Price-Pottenger Nutrition Foundation and a certified clinical nutritionist, believes that frequent consumption of common food allergens — like wheat or soy, as well as anything loaded with sugar, or anything that quickly converts into sugar (alcohol, most grains) — can promote inflammation, which wreaks havoc on the body's joints.

"We are living organisms that contain a masterful, self-healing ability," says Getoff. "If we feed our bodies the right foods and additional nutrients, our bodies can begin to heal on their own, perhaps without having to take potentially-harmful drugs."

Getoff advises eating healthily — meaning free of allergy-promoting foods — for at least two months. According to him, it takes six weeks for wheat to clear out of the system. Perhaps due to its modern, stripped-of-nutrition, hybridized ubiquity, wheat may trigger an auto-immune reaction in many people. Make sure to cut out foods that may seem more innocuous than regular table sugar but that also may promote inflammation, like fruit, honey, molasses and agave.

Do Our Smartphones Make Us Dumb?

How Much Time DO We Spend on our Smartphones?

On average, smartphone users spend between 2-4 hours every day hunched over their phones, checking email, texting, or in their apps. That's almost 1400 hours every year that people are putting their spines in a compromised position.

According to New York spine surgeon Dr. Kenneth Hansraj, "texting is like lifting weights but doing so unwittingly." He determined that, when you bend your head forward at 15 degrees, its weight effectively increases from 12 pounds to 27 pounds. At 45 degrees, your head exerts 49 pounds of force, and at 60 degrees, 60 pounds — this is like carrying an eight-year-old child around your neck for several hours a day!

The problem is really obvious in kids. Stress on their neck is leading to complaints of neck pain and headaches from smartphone users, some as young as nine years old.

Why do we compulsively do what obviously hurts us?

We Are Changing Our Neurochemistry

Compulsive texting is a very frequent disorder. In fact, 23% of teens say they send and receive over 100 messages each day. 9% say they text compulsively. That's a total of 23 out of every 100 teens saying they send and/or receive over 100 messages every day. That's a lot of messages.

Both teens and text-dependent adults are becoming even more restless, easily bored creatures and, for too many of us, our gadgets give us in abundance qualities our neurochemical systems find particularly exciting. Novelty is one.

The dopamine delivery system is activated by finding something unexpected or by the anticipation of something new. If the rewards come unpredictably — as text messages do — we get even more carried away. No wonder we called our earliest smartphones "CrackBerries."

The system is also activated by particular types of cues that a reward is coming. In order to have the maximum effect, the cues should be small, discrete, specific — like the bell Russian physiologist Ivan Pavlov rang for his dogs.

Washington State University neuroscientist Jaak Panksepp says a way to drive animals into a frenzy is to give them only tiny bits of food: This simultaneously stimulating and unsatisfying tease sends the seeking system into hyperactivity. University of Michigan professor of psychology Kent Berridge says the "ding" announcing the arrival of a text message serves as a reward cue for us. And when we respond, we get a little piece of news that makes us want more. We seek this buzz to our physical detriment.

We Are Changing Our Anatomy

Over time, this poor posture, or text neck, can lead to early wear and tear on our spines and eventually cause degeneration and arthritis regardless of age. Still, pain doesn't seem to register when we're getting the dopamine buzz of being "plugged in" to this random reward system.

Imagine if we keep up this bad habit what will happen to our posture, to our spines. The neck should have a natural reverse C-shaped curve, but patients with text neck are beginning to lose their neck's natural curve. Instead, the vertebrae in their neck are stacked on top of one another.

Without the natural curve in our spines, the joints in our neck begin to degenerate. The discs (or soft jelly-like tissue) between our vertebra eventually give out because of the pressure. This is the beginning of arthritis.

With little room for nerves to exit, they become pinched and irritated. This can cause severe neck pain, stiff neck, shoulder pain and headaches.

Do you have a phone that lets you text, surf the web, and play games? That's a lot of mileage for your thumbs. Chiropractors have begun reporting cases of arthritis at the base of the thumb in younger people, possibly related to texting.

NOTE: When your thumbs begin to ache, give the texting a rest. If pain continues, use your phone to reach out to us at Living Well Chiropractic [LivingWellBainbridge.com]. We have effective treatments for arthritis.

It's Never Too Late!

The good news? We've only been using smartphones since the 21st century, it's not too late to break these dangerous patterns. There are ways we can catch ourselves in the act of this addictive habit and switch gears. Cultivating mindfulness and choosing contrary action gives us its own neurochemical reward. We feel more confident that we are choosing what is ultimately a kinder relationship to our bodies and others,

It doesn't hurt to experiment with new behaviour. Try leaving your phone at the door when you enter your dwelling. Or if going out, try leaving it in the car. Our concentration improves as a result. When we spend time with people we may feel jittery at first, but this new practice can give us the capacity to be present, to listen better, to connect in more satisfying ways. But, like all habits, practice makes perfect (or good enough).

Chiropractic care is about treating the source of the symptoms and educating patients on new practices that will support their freedom from pain.

Don't Get Caught Off Guard: Prepare Your Kids for Success in Sports

Kids Love Team Sports

The current generation of children is more athletic than any before. In fact, it's estimated that nearly 30 million U.S. children and adolescents are active in youth sports on fields, courts and rinks each year. These young athletes are enjoying many physical, social and emotional benefits from playing sports but unfortunately, there are also risks.

The Chiropractic Connection

Participation in youth sports is not only booming, it's something children are starting at earlier ages. I know as a hockey player, I was out on the ice training as early as 5 or 6 years old. Now I know, youth sports puts young, developing structures into demand physically and opens the door for trauma." But I also know that chiropractic care can play a critical role in helping kids minimize injuries and perform at their peak. "Chiropractic's focus on the spinal structure and nervous system is so important for children since they're in growth and development stages," he says. "Chiropractors are also huge educators for parents and kids about how to optimize performance through healthy lifestyles."

Research shows there is a positive connection between chiropractic care and athleticism. A study of athletes by the Journal of Chiropractic Research and Clinical Investigation concluded that athletes who received 12 weeks of chiropractic care exhibited 30 percent improvement in reaction time versus a group with no chiropractic care. The *Journal of Vertebral Subluxation Research* shows baseball players receiving chiropractic treatments enjoyed significant improvement in their capillary count, which leads to healthy oxygenation of blood supply crucial for muscle function, performance and healing.

The Right Guidance

It's important to give kids ongoing guidance to prevent injury and enjoy a great playing experience. This means making sure they're eating healthy meals and snacks, drinking plenty of water, maintaining a proper weight and getting enough rest. Check in with your child's coach to make sure s/he is using equipment correctly and that they're warming up and cooling down properly.

Out of the many sports injuries that Living Well Chiropractic treats include:

- Achilles tendinitis
- ankle sprain
- elbow bursitis
- golfer's elbow
- groin strain
- hamstring strain
- iliotibial band syndrome (IT Band)
- low back strain

- plantar fasciitis
- rotator cuff strain

Don't hesitate to set up a general assessment for your child before the season begins. Doing so may be the best way to evaluate their form and learn new habits that will take them all the way to their "A-Game."

Staying Strong Between Sessions

Going to the chiropractor every week for the rest of your life isn't right for anyone. It would be time consuming, costly and just, plain silly. But, after an adjustment, you just feel so good! Your joints are more lubricated. Your muscles are less tense, and you finally have more energy to do what you love!

But, over time, your spine can settle back into its old pattern, especially if your habits of standing and sitting remain the same. The truism is right: Nothing changes if nothing changes.

So, what steps can you take to extend the time between your chiropractic adjustments?

Be Patient

Healing is a process. The damage to your spine and joints didn't happen overnight. The healing process will also take time. Luckily, each visit builds on the one before, and each adjustment will last longer than the prior one. Once you finish your treatment plan, your muscles will be realigned.

Stay Active

Avoid sitting for a long period of time immediately following your chiropractic adjustment. Your adjustment restores motion and frees locked up areas of the spine. Make the most of this fact. If you can do it that day, go for a walk even if it's just to the mailbox. If you're recovering from a specific injury, ask your chiropractor for exercises that specifically address that area of the body, and keep your commitment to your change by doing them.

Stay Hydrated

You should drink half your body weight in ounces. If you weigh 160 pounds, drink at least 80 ounces of water each day.

Sleep Well

We spend 7-9 hours each night sleeping. Choose a pillow that conforms to the curve in your neck. Ordinary pillows are all one height. This puts pressure on your neck as you sleep — especially back-sleepers. The right pillow is important.

At Living Well, we make available *ChiroFlow* — our favorite water-based pillow for interested patients! They are thicker on one side and allow your head to drop down on the other. This makes your head even with your shoulders. Your chiropractor may also have suggestions for good pillows. Sleep position matters as well. If you have sleep apnea, arthritis or injury, changing your nightly habits may give you relief.

Sit Upright

If you're sitting at a computer, adjust it so your eyes stare mid-screen. If you look up or down, neck and shoulder trouble will follow. Your elbows should be to your side at a 90-degree angle and your wrists should be supported by a wrist rest. If you use a mouse, be sure it is within reach. Positioning your body correctly can minimize muscle strain and help you maintain your alignment.

Fix Your Rear-View Mirror

After your chiropractic adjustment, position your rear-view mirror so you can see clearly. Then, the next time you get in, don't adjust the mirror. Adjust your body position. This will help you to keep up proper posture while driving.

How Often Must I See a Chiropractor?

Remember that you are a body in motion! Your visits to the chiropractor make up a tiny, tiny, fraction of time in your week. The real work is happening all around you, at all times. Your body is constantly remodeling, regenerating, and responding to its environment, inside and out. Being aware of your body posture and joint position is an essential component to reaching your maximum benefit from your chiropractic care. Ask yourself how many hours a day you spend working? How many days a year are spent in the repetitive motion of your occupation? How many days a week are you active and exerting yourself?

When you begin to comprehend the way the body structures develop and modify with usage over time, you can start to answer the question, HOW often should I be adjusted?

Keeping Fit for Top Performance

Keeping fit is vital to success in any sport. Sometimes training too hard can give athletes trouble whether it's a sprained ankle, golf/tennis-elbow, a torn rotator cuff or what's called a stinger. Being stopped by physical pain can become a nightmare. Some athletes try to enhance performance by using drugs to treat an injury, so they can still stay in the game, but most look to nutrition, workouts, and regular practice as methods to get better. One way athletes can improve is through chiropractic care.

Get Back Out There

Chiropractic care helps athletes both prevent and recover from injuries. Spinal adjustments can align your vertebrae, so your tendons and muscles heal properly. If you're experiencing stubborn pain from a past injury that won't seem to heal, chiropractic care can get to the root of the injury and correct the problem at its source, so your symptoms lessen or disappear.

With improved strength, balance, stability, flexibility and range of motion, you'll notice improved performance with regular chiropractic treatment. We find *if you listen to your body when it whispers, you won't have to hear it scream.*

Expect Improvement

How an athlete improves with chiropractic is by taking pressure off nerves in the spinal column. When your spinal vertebrae are misaligned, the impulses sent from your brain to parts of your body through your spine may not be as clear as they should be. When these impulses are restricted, your body can shut down or contract to protect itself from further injury— this is an involuntary instinct. When we constrict movement, we will not be operating at full capacity, and your athletic performance can suffer.

If you want an edge in your game, try chiropractic treatment and see if it helps. Once the pathways between your brain and muscles, heart and lungs are clear, you'll be amazed at what you can do.

Chiropractic Care May Help Us Stay Fit

Every week that goes by, seems there's at least one fad diet that comes down the pike. Whether it's recommended by Dr. Oz, pitched to us from magazines in the grocery checkout, or merely blasted at us over social media, we at Living Well believe these extreme diets — like the weight loss they promise — come as fast as they go.

Americans suffer from a national eating disorder: our unhealthy obsession with yo-yo dieting (stuffing or starving), keeps us out of balance. Snowballing rates of obesity, diabetes, and heart disease can be traced to our unhealthy diets. So how do we change?

The weight loss industry is a 40 billion dollar one and continues to grow because almost all of us in the "first world" have been raised to doubt our value if we don't look like hot actors or young models who live on kale. Thus, many of us, especially women (the target market), have a love-hate relationship with our bodies and the foods we eat. While there is no magic potion to imbibe to return our bodies and minds to balance, there are many natural options available for cultivating a better lifestyle.

At Living Well, we say, "Don't believe anything the diet industry tells you!" Why? Because their job isn't to tell the truth — it's to make money. They are allowed to lie; these companies make their money off failure, not success. They need you to fail at weight loss, so you'll pay them again for an easy fix. It's like any Casino; one-time customers are not the sort of thing that keep these companies in business.

Most nutrition and obesity studies have found that the safest bet to reaching and maintaining a physically healthy body is to consume less and exercise more — not through starving, juicing, renouncing fat and carbs, or working out like a weekend warrior but by caring for yourself as a way of life.

As scientist Michael Pollan says, "Eat food, not too much, mostly plants."

Probably the first two words are most important. "Eat food" means to eat real food — vegetables, fruits, whole grains, and, yes, fish and meat — and to avoid what Pollan calls "edible food-like substances," those manufactured "foods" you have to unwrap from their packages. Another truism: If it doesn't rot within a week or your great grandmother couldn't find it in her home, it's toxic no matter how many times the word Natural is written on its packaging.

Many of us need to change other things too, like the ways we live, our attitude towards our bodies, the ways we move and how we pace ourselves in our daily lives. But, did you know that chiropractic care can promote and help you maintain balanced weight loss?

Although chiropractic is great for correcting any misalignments in the spine, your chiropractor is a great resource for overall body wellness. At Living Well, we understand that everything in the body is connected. It's important to make sure your entire body, and your relationship to it, is healthy, not just visually thinner.

If you're not connected to your body's experience, you'll never treat it right. No matter how much weight you lose on a magic-bullet diet, science shows you'll gain it back plus more. If what you put into your body changes but nothing else does, that physical shift won't last.

Our staff at Living Well can offer nutritional counselling and wellness guidance for each individual patient. We do this is by evaluating your current lifestyle and by co-creating a plan with you that is suited for your particular needs, ability and preferences.

By functioning as your allies and holding you accountable to your new practices, steady progress is inevitable. Studies show that those who implement a multi-faceted health program usually see better and lasting results.

What is probably news to you is that by receiving regular adjustments, healthy weight loss goals can be achieved (at least according to recent studies). When pressure is taken off the spine, a person is more flexible and better able to exercise without pain or discomfort.

By having a spine free of subluxations, stress hormones like adrenaline, cortisol, norepinephrine won't need to saturate your body with a "shut down" response; a pattern that creates not only stress, sleep deprivation/exhaustion but a sluggish metabolism. Experts agree, when you're not balanced, you are more likely to shovel in quick energy, chemically-manufactured, high-sugar foods and skip workouts. When amped up or exhausted (same hormonal coin), who wants to eat whole foods, move more intentionally, or even workout?

Adrenaline, Cortisol, Norepinephrine are the three major stress hormones that insure fad diets won't work.

Visiting your chiropractor regularly and receiving adjustments, can also be restorative after a workout. Many patients feel and sleep much better and even breathe more deeply following an adjustment. Chiropractic and nutritional care at Living Well may also keep you motivated and strong for your next workout. As you gain traction in your healthier lifestyle, you feel better about yourself. With more confidence, you're more likely to maintain your progress.

As a chiropractor and an active athlete, I see to it that no patient's injuries go unnoticed. If you use improper form when jogging, climbing or working out, you open yourself up to destructive patterns, ones you might miss. I have a hawk's eye in this regard and can usually decipher bad habits that lead to possible injuries. I won't hesitate to advise you on proper form and remind you about how important it is to take care of your body in a holistic way.

As we all now agree, diets don't work especially if they're too restrictive, tasteless and require joyless exercise routines. If you're not enlivened in your body, mind and soul, you won't stand a chance. As fitness guru Richard Simmons says, "There's a reason the first three letters in diet spell DIE." But with changing up your self-care regimens and engaging in steady chiropractic care, you can achieve and maintain your health goals. Returning to the vibrant body you've always wanted takes time and effort, but by taking advantage of all that supports you, it is possible.

~

Life is not merely about living, but about living well!

ABOUT THE AUTHOR

Dr. Brian Kovara graduated from Northwestern College of Chiropractic in 2000 but his vision to improve the quality of life for others began much earlier. Dr. Kovara is fond of working with families and continues to grow professionally in the fields of sports medicine, spinal decompression, pediatrics, and nutrition. His wife April Blanchard Kovara and his three kids cherish living and playing in the Pacific Northwest.